Oral Health and Environmentally Related Factors Associated with General Health and Quality of Life

Oral Health and Environmentally Related Factors Associated with General Health and Quality of Life

Editors

Gaetano Isola
Romeo Patini

MDPI • Basel • Beijing • Wuhan • Barcelona • Belgrade • Manchester • Tokyo • Cluj • Tianjin

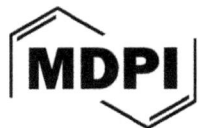

Editors
Gaetano Isola
University of Catania
Italy

Romeo Patini
Università Cattolica del Sacro Cuore
Italy

Editorial Office
MDPI
St. Alban-Anlage 66
4052 Basel, Switzerland

This is a reprint of articles from the Special Issue published online in the open access journal *Applied Sciences* (ISSN 2076-3417) (available at: https://www.mdpi.com/journal/applsci/special_issues/Oral_Health_Life).

For citation purposes, cite each article independently as indicated on the article page online and as indicated below:

LastName, A.A.; LastName, B.B.; LastName, C.C. Article Title. *Journal Name* **Year**, *Article Number*, Page Range.

ISBN 978-3-03936-858-7 (Hbk)
ISBN 978-3-03936-859-4 (PDF)

© 2020 by the authors. Articles in this book are Open Access and distributed under the Creative Commons Attribution (CC BY) license, which allows users to download, copy and build upon published articles, as long as the author and publisher are properly credited, which ensures maximum dissemination and a wider impact of our publications.

The book as a whole is distributed by MDPI under the terms and conditions of the Creative Commons license CC BY-NC-ND.

Contents

About the Editors vii

Gaetano Isola
Oral Health and Related Factors Associated with General Health and Quality of Life
Reprinted from: *Appl. Sci.* **2020**, *10*, 4663, doi:10.3390/app10134663 1

Rosa Valletta, Ada Pango, Gregorio Tortora, Roberto Rongo, Vittorio Simeon, Gianrico Spagnuolo and Vincenzo D'Antò
Association between Gingival Biotype and Facial Typology through Cephalometric Evaluation and Three-Dimensional Facial Scanning
Reprinted from: *Appl. Sci.* **2019**, *9*, 5057, doi:10.3390/app9235057 7

Mario Dioguardi, Vito Crincoli, Luigi Laino, Mario Alovisi, Enrica Laneve, Diego Sovereto, Bruna Raddato, Khrystyna Zhurakivska, Filiberto Mastrangelo, Domenico Ciavarella, Lucio Lo Russo and Lorenzo Lo Muzio
Surface Alterations Induced on Endodontic Instruments by Sterilization Processes, Analyzed with Atomic Force Microscopy: A Systematic Review
Reprinted from: *Appl. Sci.* **2019**, *9*, 4948, doi:10.3390/app9224948 19

Alessandro Polizzi, Salvatore Torrisi, Simona Santonocito, Mattia Di Stefano, Francesco Indelicato and Antonino Lo Giudice
Influence of Myeloperoxidase Levels on Periodontal Disease: An Applied Clinical Study
Reprinted from: *Appl. Sci.* **2020**, *10*, 1037, doi:10.3390/app10031037 35

Antonino Lo Giudice, Gaetano Isola, Lorenzo Rustico, Vincenzo Ronsivalle, Marco Portelli and Riccardo Nucera
The Efficacy of Retention Appliances after Fixed Orthodontic Treatment: A Systematic Review and Meta-Analysis
Reprinted from: *Appl. Sci.* **2020**, *10*, 3107, doi:10.3390/app10093107 49

Soo Hwan Byun, Chanyang Min, Yong Bok Kim, Heejin Kim, Sung Hun Kang, Bum Jung Park, Ji Hye Wee, Hyo Geun Choi and Seok Jin Hong
Analysis of Chronic Periodontitis in Tonsillectomy Patients: A Longitudinal Follow-Up Study Using a National Health Screening Cohort
Reprinted from: *Appl. Sci.* **2020**, *10*, 3663, doi:10.3390/app10103663 65

João Albernaz Neves, Nathalie Antunes-Ferreira, Vanessa Machado, João Botelho, Luís Proença, Alexandre Quintas, José João Mendes and Ana Sintra Delgado
Sex Prediction Based on Mesiodistal Width Data in the Portuguese Population
Reprinted from: *Appl. Sci.* **2020**, *10*, 4156, doi:10.3390/app10124156 75

Dinis Pereira, Vanessa Machado, João Botelho, Luís Proença, José João Mendes and Ana Sintra Delgado
Comparison of Pain Perception between Clear Aligners and Fixed Appliances: A Systematic Review and Meta-Analysis
Reprinted from: *Appl. Sci.* **2020**, *10*, 4276, doi:10.3390/app10124276 - 83

About the Editors

Gaetano Isola is Assistant Professor at the University of Catania, Catania, Italy. Qualified in Dentistry in 2009 at the University of Messina, Italy. He completed his Ph.D. in "Physiopathology of the Stomatognathic Apparatus and Dental Materials" at the University of Turin, Turin, Italy. He was a visiting Research Fellow at the "Laboratory the Study of Calcified Tissues and Biomaterials" at the Department of Periodontology Université de Montréal, Canada, Advanced Course in Periodontology at the University of Ferrara, the Master Course in Periodontology at the University of Verona, and the Three-year certificate in Oral Surgery at the University of Naples "Federico II". He was a Visiting Professor at the Department of Periodontology at the University of North Carolina at Chapel Hill, USA and the Department of Oral Surgery of the University of Granada, Spain. He was a Visiting Researcher at the Department of Implantology and Oral Surgery at the University of Bern, Switzerland, and the Department of Periodontology of the "Eastman Dental Institute", London. He was also National Scientific Qualification of Associate Professor for the Academic Discipline of Odontostomatology, Sector 06/F1, Italian Minister of University and Research (MIUR). Dr. Isola has been a recipient of many research awards, among others the "Global Peer Review Awards" of the Web of Science Group, the Travel Grant Award 2020" and "Outstanding Reviewer Award 2019" from MDPI Publishing and selected for the "IADR Robert Frank Junior Award" CED-IADR/NOF Oral Health Research Association and the "USERN 2020 award", Universal Scientific Education and Research Network (USERN). He is an active member of the Italian Society of Oral Surgery (SIdCO) and the International Piezoelectric Surgery Academy (IPA). Board of the International Association of Dental Research (IADR) and a member of the Italian Society of Periodontology (SIdP). He is also an active member of the "International IADR Constitution Committee" of the International Association of Dental Research (IADR) (2016-2019), and 2019-2022. He has served as an advisor for several research projects and a speaker at national and international conferences of Periodontology and Oral Surgery. He is an author of over 100 national and international peer-reviewed publications. His main research interests focus on the clinical, biological, and pharmacological aspects of periodontitis, and the relationship between oral health and systemic health.

Romeo Patini is Assistant Professor at the University of Sacred Heart of Rome, Rome, Italy. Graduated in Dentistry at the Catholic University of the Sacred Heart in Rome in 2011, he got a Post-Graduate Diploma in Oral Surgery at "Sapienza – University of Rome" and a Ph.D. in Clinical, Cellular, and Molecular Research in Dentistry at the Catholic University of Sacred Heart in Rome in 2017. Since April 1st, 2018, he has been a Research Fellow at the same University in which he graduated. His areas of expertise include periodontology, implantology, oral microbiota, and connections between oral and systemic diseases. His interests also include research methodology, and, particularly, systematic reviews and meta-analyses. He is the author of more than 100 contributions (including scientific articles, abstracts, and posters) in national and international peer-reviewed journals. He has been an invited speaker at various national and international dentistry congresses.

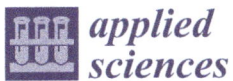

Editorial

Oral Health and Related Factors Associated with General Health and Quality of Life

Gaetano Isola

Department of General Surgery and Surgical-Medical Specialties, School of Dentistry, University of Catania, 95124 Catania, Italy; gaetano.isola@unict.it; Tel.: +39-095-3782453

Received: 30 May 2020; Accepted: 25 June 2020; Published: 6 July 2020

Abstract: Oral well-being is an integral part of individual general health. The mouth and teeth are, in fact, part of our body, increasingly characterizing personal identity. Oral diseases are a public health problem that has a growing prevalence. Oral pathologies can occur in childhood, and as they have a chronic and progressive course, if not properly treated, they can affect the relational, psychological, and social skills of an individual. The population most affected are those with a low socio-economic level, so much so that the presence of diseases of the oral cavity is considered a marker of social disadvantage. In this regard, much effort is needed from scientists, and their applied sciences, in order to give the knowledge required for public health personal to take note of the seriousness of the situation and to start changing the way we deal with the problem.

Keywords: oral health; periodontitis; systemic health; caries; oral pathology; applied sciences

1. Editorial

In July 2019, The Lancet published a full-bodied report: "Oral diseases: a global public health challenge" dedicated to investigating this topic, often overlooked by public health policies [1]. The relationship is the result of a collaboration between thirteen world academic institutions. Top experts in the field of preventive and community dentistry took part in the work. Many of them are part of the WHO collaboration centers for oral health inequalities. In this work the main pathologies of the hard and soft tissues of the oral cavity were analyzed, from which the different chapters of the relationship derive: (1) Overview of oral pathologies, (2) Epidemiology, (3) Effects at the individual, family and social level, and (4) Social determinants ampersands.

1.1. Caries

Caries is a chronic-degenerative pathology with a multifactorial etiology resulting from alternation of periods of demineralization and re-mineralization linked to the pH of the bacterial plaque [2,3].

The reduction in pH is due to the presence of acidogenic and aciduric bacteria that ferment sugars taken in through the diet. A cavitary lesion is the clinical sign of caries disease, which can be arrested in its early stages through correct exposure to fluorinated compounds [4]. Fluorine is the cornerstone of caries prevention and is necessary for all individuals with natural dental elements [5]. It is also important to obtain a good endodontic treatment in cases of endodontic lesions. In this regard, Dioguardi et al., in their systematic review published in the present Special Issue, have underlined the importance of the sterilization process of endodontic instruments as a key factor for an endodontic treatment [6].

1.2. Periodontal Disease

Periodontitis is a chronic inflammatory disease of the supporting tissues of the dental elements caused by the presence of anaerobic bacteria with the interaction of three main cofactors: host susceptibility, environmental, and behavioral factors [7–11]. More specifically, Valletta et al. [12] have evaluated the association between facial typology and gingival biotype in patients by means of two-dimensional and three-dimensional evaluations of facial typology using facial scanners. The authors found that there was no statistically significant association between facial typology and gingival biotype. Polizzi et al., in their report, have underlined the fundamental role of Myeloperoxidase in the alveolar bone loss during periodontitis [13], while Byun et al. have shown the role exerted of periodontitis in patients that undergo tonsillectomy [14].

Tobacco and chronic diseases such as diabetes, cardiovascular disease, and dementia contribute to increased risk of periodontal disease. The disease manifests itself in its initial stage as gingivitis, a reversible pathology characterized by bleeding, swelling of the gums, edema, and the absence of periodontal pockets [15,16]. If left untreated, it develops into periodontitis, an irreversible pathology characterized by radiographic loss of bone in the presence of loss of attachment to the probe [17] is a pathognomonic sign of the periodontal pocket [18,19], especially during orthodontic treatment, as shown by Lo Giudice et al. in their report [20].

1.3. Oral Cancer

Oral cancer in all its forms (e.g., carcinoma of the lip, tongue, pharynx, and oral cavity) is increasingly common worldwide [1,21]. Squamous cell carcinoma is the most common cancer in the oral cavity [22]. The main risk factors are smoking and tobacco, especially if chewed (in the form of Bethel leaves), alcohol, and infectious agents. The most affected demographic is that of elderly men of low socio-economic level. Oral papilloma caused by Human Papillomaviruses (HPV) is particularly frequent in high-income populations, especially among younger demographics.

2. Epidemiology of Oral Pathologies

The latest epidemiological studies reveal that data on caries not treated with deciduous and permanent dentition have remained unchanged over the past 30 years, to the detriment of what is perceived by academic and non-academic society. Data from 2017 confirm that untreated caries in permanent teeth remain the most common disease worldwide, affecting 34.1% of the population [1] (Figure 1).

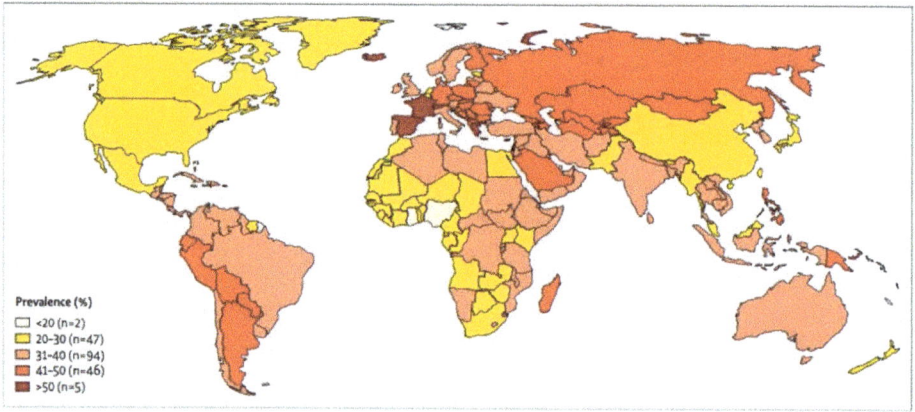

Figure 1. World prevalence estimate of untreated caries in permanent dentition in 2017, from the Institute of Health Metrics and Evaluation.

Despite the undoubted improvements obtained in terms of general health, the incidence of various pathologies of dental interest remains high.

It is, therefore, necessary to promote and favor specific caries prevention programs for periodontal diseases and neoplasms in order also to avoid the onset of clinical conditions that entail disabling psychophysical impairments, with a consequent commitment of substantial financial, personal, and collective resources for rehabilitation therapy [23,24].

The etiology, pathogenesis, and evolution of the aforementioned pathologies, and the fact that prevention represents a fundamental measure in terms of efficacy and favorable cost-benefit ratio, are well known.

Furthermore, since various risk factors for diseases of the oral cavity (e.g., bacteria, inadequate diet, smoking, incorrect lifestyle) are common to other chronic degenerative diseases, any preventive measure put in place must be considered as a wider measure of promotion of individual overall health [25].

Most of the most common pathologies of the oral cavity, for diagnostic purposes [26], make use of well-coded and proven efficacy pathways, ranging from general medical anamnesis to specific stomatological anamnesis [27], to extra-intra-oral physical examination [28], to radiographic investigations, photographic documentation, and examination of study models [29–33]. Furthermore, the introduction to daily practice of recent innovative technologies will allow clinicians to obtain increasingly precise and punctual information, in order to considerably reduce the margin of diagnostic error.

The overall disease burden of oral disease, understood as a measure of the weight of the disease according to the disability-adjusted life year (DALY) index, is comparable to that of tuberculosis or malaria [30].

Here then, is the paradox of oral health: In the face of a very high number of affected individuals, of the sufferings and consequences of oral diseases on general health [34–38], which are moreover particularly serious in children, the underestimation of the problem appears scandalous.

3. Conclusions

Therefore, the time has come for public health to take note of the seriousness of the situation and to start changing the way we deal with the problem. It is possible to improve oral health and reduce inequalities at a global level by investing resources in prevention and basic care, and not by relying exclusively on the private dentistry market, which can be accessed by a dramatically low number of people compared to the many who need it.

Author Contributions: Conceptualization, validation, writing—review and editing, G.I. The author has read and agreed to the published version of the manuscript.

Funding: This research received no external funding.

Conflicts of Interest: The author declares no conflict of interest.

References

1. Peres, M.A.; Macpherson, L.M.D.; Weyant, R.J.; Daly, B.; Venturelli, R.; Mathur, M.R.; Listl, S.; Celeste, R.K.; Guarnizo-Herreno, C.C.; Kearns, C.; et al. Oral diseases: A global public health challenge. *Lancet* **2019**, *394*, 249–260. [CrossRef]
2. Yeung, A.W.K.; Jacobs, R.; Bornstein, M.M. Novel low-dose protocols using cone beam computed tomography in dental medicine: A review focusing on indications, limitations, and future possibilities. *Clin. Oral Investig.* **2019**, *23*, 2573–2581. [CrossRef]
3. Aarabi, G.; Heydecke, G.; Seedorf, U. Roles of Oral Infections in the Pathomechanism of Atherosclerosis. *Int. J. Mol. Sci.* **2018**, *19*, 1978. [CrossRef]
4. Patini, R.; Cattani, P.; Marchetti, S.; Isola, G.; Quaranta, G.; Gallenzi, P. Evaluation of Predation Capability of Periodontopathogens Bacteria by Bdellovibrio Bacteriovorus HD100. An in Vitro Study. *Materials* **2019**, *12*, 208. [CrossRef] [PubMed]

5. Iram, S.; Zahera, M.; Wahid, I.; Baker, A.; Raish, M.; Khan, A.; Ali, N.; Ahmad, S.; Khan, M.S. Cisplatin bioconjugated enzymatic GNPs amplify the effect of cisplatin with acquiescence. *Sci. Rep.* **2019**, *9*, 13826. [CrossRef]
6. Dioguardi, M.; Crincoli, V.; Laino, L.; Alovisi, M.; Laneve, E.; Sovereto, D.; Raddato, B.; Zhurakivska, K.; Mastrangelo, F.; Ciavarella, D.; et al. Surface Alterations Induced on Endodontic Instruments by Sterilization Processes, Analyzed with Atomic Force Microscopy: A Systematic Review. *Appl. Sci.* **2019**, *9*, 4948. [CrossRef]
7. Isola, G.; Giudice, A.L.; Polizzi, A.; Alibrandi, A.; Patini, R.; Ferlito, S. Periodontitis and Tooth Loss Have Negative Systemic Impact on Circulating Progenitor Cell Levels: A Clinical Study. *Genes* **2019**, *10*, 1022. [CrossRef]
8. Isola, G.; Polizzi, A.; Iorio-Siciliano, V.; Alibrandi, A.; Ramaglia, L.; Leonardi, R. Effectiveness of a nutraceutical agent in the non-surgical periodontal therapy: A randomized, controlled clinical trial. *Clin. Oral Investig.* **2020**. [CrossRef]
9. Isola, G.; Matarese, G.; Ramaglia, L.; Pedulla, E.; Rapisarda, E.; Iorio-Siciliano, V. Association between periodontitis and glycosylated haemoglobin before diabetes onset: A cross-sectional study. *Clin. Oral Investig.* **2019**. [CrossRef]
10. Isola, G.; Polizzi, A.; Santonocito, S.; Alibrandi, A.; Ferlito, S. Expression of Salivary and Serum Malondialdehyde and Lipid Profile of Patients with Periodontitis and Coronary Heart Disease. *Int. J. Mol. Sci.* **2019**, *20*, 6061. [CrossRef]
11. Isola, G.; Alibrandi, A.; Curro, M.; Matarese, M.; Ricca, S.; Matarese, G.; Ientile, R.; Kocher, T. Evaluation of salivary and serum ADMA levels in patients with periodontal and cardiovascular disease as subclinical marker of cardiovascular risk. *J. Periodontol.* **2020**. [CrossRef]
12. Valletta, R.; Pango, A.; Tortora, G.; Rongo, R.; Simeon, V.; Spagnuolo, G.; D'Anto, V. Association between Gingival Biotype and Facial Typology through Cephalometric Evaluation and Three-Dimensional Facial Scanning. *Appl. Sci.* **2019**, *9*. [CrossRef]
13. Polizzi, A.; Torrisi, S.; Santonocito, S.; Di Stefano, M.; Indelicato, F.; Lo Giudice, A. Influence of Myeloperoxidase Levels on Periodontal Disease: An Applied Clinical Study. *Appl. Sci.* **2020**, *10*, 1037. [CrossRef]
14. Byun, S.H.; Min, C.; Kim, Y.B.; Kim, H.; Kang, S.H.; Park, B.J.; Wee, J.H.; Choi, H.G.; Hong, S.J. Analysis of Chronic Periodontitis in Tonsillectomy Patients: A Longitudinal Follow-Up Study Using a National Health Screening Cohort. *Appl. Sci.* **2020**, *10*, 3663. [CrossRef]
15. Isola, G.; Alibrandi, A.; Rapisarda, E.; Matarese, G.; Williams, R.C.; Leonardi, R. Association of vitamin D in patients with periodontitis: A cross-sectional study. *J. Periodontal Res.* **2020**. [CrossRef]
16. Isola, G.; Polizzi, A.; Alibrandi, A.; Indelicato, F.; Ferlito, S. Analysis of Endothelin-1 Concentrations in Individuals with Periodontitis. *Sci. Rep.* **2020**, *10*, 1652. [CrossRef]
17. Patini, R.; Coviello, V.; Riminucci, M.; Corsi, A.; Cicconetti, A. Early-stage diffuse large B-cell lymphoma of the submental region: A case report and review of the literature. *Oral Surgery* **2017**, *10*, 56–60. [CrossRef]
18. Facciolo, M.T.; Riva, F.; Gallenzi, P.; Patini, R.; Gaglioti, D. A rare case of oral multisystem Langerhans cell histiocytosis. *J. Clin. Exp. Dent.* **2017**, *9*, e820–e824. [CrossRef]
19. Martellacci, L.; Quaranta, G.; Patini, R.; Isola, G.; Gallenzi, P.; Masucci, L. A Literature Review of Metagenomics and Culturomics of the Peri-implant Microbiome: Current Evidence and Future Perspectives. *Materials* **2019**, *12*, 3010. [CrossRef]
20. Lo Giudice, A.; Isola, G.; Rustico, L.; Ronsivalle, V.; Portelli, M.; Nucera, R. The Efficacy of Retention Appliances after Fixed Orthodontic Treatment: A Systematic Review and Meta-Analysis. *Appl. Sci.* **2020**, *10*, 3107. [CrossRef]
21. Suez, J.; Zmora, N.; Segal, E.; Elinav, E. The pros, cons, and many unknowns of probiotics. *Nat. Med.* **2019**, *25*, 716–729. [CrossRef]
22. Patini, R.; Staderini, E.; Gallenzi, P. Multidisciplinary surgical management of Cowden syndrome: Report of a case. *J. Clin. Exp. Dent.* **2016**, *18*, 472–474. [CrossRef] [PubMed]
23. Pelo, S.; Saponaro, G.; Patini, R.; Staderini, E.; Giordano, A.; Gasparini, G.; Garagiola, U.; Azzuni, C.; Cordaro, M.; Foresta, E.; et al. Risks in surgery-first orthognathic approach: Complications of segmental osteotomies of the jaws. A systematic review. *Eur. Rev. Med. Pharmacol. Sci.* **2017**, *21*, 4–12. [PubMed]

24. Patini, R.; Arrica, M.; Di Stasio, E.; Gallenzi, P.; Cordaro, M. The use of magnetic resonance imaging in the evaluation of upper airway structures in paediatric obstructive sleep apnoea syndrome: A systematic review and meta-analysis. *Dentomaxillofacial Radiol.* **2016**, *45*, 20160136. [CrossRef]
25. Arweiler, N.B.; Marx, V.K.; Laugisch, O.; Sculean, A.; Auschill, T.M. Clinical evaluation of a newly developed chairside test to determine periodontal pathogens. *J. Periodontol.* **2020**, *91*, 387–395. [CrossRef] [PubMed]
26. Isola, G.; Matarese, M.; Ramaglia, L.; Cicciu, M.; Matarese, G. Evaluation of the efficacy of celecoxib and ibuprofen on postoperative pain, swelling, and mouth opening after surgical removal of impacted third molars: A randomized, controlled clinical trial. *Int. J. Oral Maxillofac. Surg.* **2019**, *48*, 1348–1354. [CrossRef]
27. Isola, G.; Alibrandi, A.; Pedulla, E.; Grassia, V.; Ferlito, S.; Perillo, L.; Rapisarda, E. Analysis of the Effectiveness of Lornoxicam and Flurbiprofen on Management of Pain and Sequelae Following Third Molar Surgery: A Randomized, Controlled, Clinical Trial. *J. Clin. Med.* **2019**, *8*, 325. [CrossRef]
28. Lo Giudice, A.; Ortensi, L.; Farronato, M.; Lucchese, A.; Lo Castro, E.; Isola, G. The step further smile virtual planning: Milled versus prototyped mock-ups for the evaluation of the designed smile characteristics. *BMC Oral Health.* **2020**, *20*, 165. [CrossRef]
29. Isola, G.; Perillo, L.; Migliorati, M.; Matarese, M.; Dalessandri, D.; Grassia, V.; Alibrandi, A.; Matarese, G. The impact of temporomandibular joint arthritis on functional disability and global health in patients with juvenile idiopathic arthritis. *Eur. J. Orthod.* **2019**, *41*, 117–124. [CrossRef]
30. Isola, G.; Anastasi, G.P.; Matarese, G.; Williams, R.C.; Cutroneo, G.; Bracco, P.; Piancino, M.G. Functional and molecular outcomes of the human masticatory muscles. *Oral Dis.* **2018**, *24*, 1428–1441. [CrossRef]
31. Pippi, R.; Santoro, M.; Patini, R. The central odontogenic fibroma: How difficult can be making a preliminary diagnosis. *J. Clin. Exp. Dent.* **2016**, *8*, e223–e225. [CrossRef]
32. Coviello, V.; Dehkhargani, Z.S.; Patini, R.; Cicconetti, A. Surgical ciliated cyst 12 years after Le Fort I maxillary advancement osteotomy: A case report and review of the literature. *Oral Surgery* **2017**, *10*, 165–170. [CrossRef]
33. Rosa, M.; Quinzi, V.; Marzo, G. Paediatric Orthodontics Part 1: Anterior open bite in the mixed dentition. *Eur. J. Paediatr. Dent.* **2019**, *20*, 80–82.
34. Ferro, R.; Besostri, A.; Olivieri, A.; Quinzi, V.; Scibetta, D. Prevalence of cross-bite in a sample of Italian preschoolers. *Eur. J. Paediatr. Dent.* **2016**, *17*, 307–309.
35. Neves, J.A.; Antunes-Ferreira, N.; Machado, V.; Botelho, J.; Proença, L.; Quintas, A.; Mendes, J.J.; Delgado, A.S. Sex Prediction Based on Mesiodistal Width Data in the Portuguese Population. *Appl. Sci.* **2020**, *10*, 4156. [CrossRef]
36. Pereira, D.; Machado, V.; Botelho, J.; Proença, L.; Mendes, J.J.; Delgado, A.S. Comparison of Pain Perception between Clear Aligners and Fixed Appliances: A Systematic Review and Meta-Analysis. *Appl. Sci.* **2020**, *10*, 4276. [CrossRef]
37. Tukov, A.R.; Shafranskii, I.L. Evaluating relative risk of morbidity or mortality for persons who participated in the clean-up of the Chernobyl accident (based on the DALY index). *Meditsina Truda I Promyshlennaia Ekologiia* **2001**, *2*, 24–29.
38. Kikuchi, K.; Furukawa, Y.; Tuot, S.; Pal, K.; Huot, C.; Yi, S. Association of oral health status with the CD4+ cell count in children living with HIV in Phnom Penh, Cambodia. *Sci. Rep.* **2019**, *9*, 14610. [CrossRef]

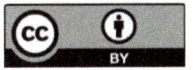

© 2020 by the author. Licensee MDPI, Basel, Switzerland. This article is an open access article distributed under the terms and conditions of the Creative Commons Attribution (CC BY) license (http://creativecommons.org/licenses/by/4.0/).

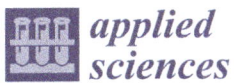

Article

Association between Gingival Biotype and Facial Typology through Cephalometric Evaluation and Three-Dimensional Facial Scanning

Rosa Valletta [1], Ada Pango [1], Gregorio Tortora [1], Roberto Rongo [1], Vittorio Simeon [2], Gianrico Spagnuolo [1,*] and Vincenzo D'Antò [1]

[1] Department of Neurosciences, Reproductive Sciences and Oral Sciences, Section of Orthodontics, University of Naples "Federico II", 80131 Naples, Italy; valletta@unina.it (R.V.); apangom@gmail.com (A.P.); gregorio.tortora@gmail.com (G.T.); roberto.rongo@gmail.com (R.R.); vincenzodanto@gmail.com (V.D.)
[2] Department of Mental Health and Preventive Medicine, Medical Statistics Unit, University of Campania "Luigi Vanvitelli", 80138 Napoli, Italy; vittoriosimeon@gmail.com
* Correspondence: gspagnuo@unina.it; Tel.: +39-081-746-2080

Received: 21 October 2019; Accepted: 21 November 2019; Published: 23 November 2019

Featured Application: Patients with a reduced inferior facial height present, with lower frequency, a thin gingival biotype, and might be less susceptible to periodontal damage due to orthodontic treatment.

Abstract: In dentistry, the assessment of periodontal biotype is considered one of the most important parameters with which to plan treatment, and craniofacial morphology might affect it. The aim of this study was to investigate the association between facial typology and gingival biotype in patients by means of two-dimensional and three-dimensional evaluations of facial typology. This study included 121 participants searching for orthodontic treatment (43 M, 78 F; 20.4 ± 10.4). Gingival biotype was evaluated based on the transparency of the periodontal probe through the gingival margin of the mid-buccal sulcus for both upper (UGB) and lower (LGB) anterior teeth. SellionNasion^GonionGnation (SN^GoGn) and CondylionGonionMenton (CoGoMe^) angles were measured on two-dimensional cephalograms. Three-dimensional face scans were acquired by means of a three-dimensional facial scanner (3dMD system) and successively analyzed to assess the facial typology using the ratio between lower facial height (SNMe) and total facial height (NMe). A chi-squared test and regression analysis were used to evaluate the associations between gingival biotype and facial morphology ($p < 0.05$). The chi-squared test showed that there was no statistically significant association between facial typology and gingival biotype (UGB $p = 0.83$; LGB $p = 0.75$). The logistic regression showed an association between SNMe/NMe and the UGB ($p = 0.036$), and SNMe/NMe and LGB ($p = 0.049$). The decreased ratio of SNMe/NMe might be a protective factor for a thin gingival biotype.

Keywords: facial typology; gingival biotype; orthodontic diagnosis; cephalometric analysis; three-dimensional facial scans

1. Introduction

Gingivitis develops more frequently in patients undergoing orthodontic treatment mainly due to an inflammatory reaction following the accumulation of bacterial plaque [1–3].

Many authors have shown that gingival recessions can develop during or after orthodontic treatment [4,5]. Indeed, at the end of orthodontic therapy, the reported prevalence of gingival recessions ranges from 5% to 12% and in long-term follow-up (5 years) has been observed an increase to 47% [4–6].

A recent systematic review has established that the direction of dental movements and the buccal-lingual thickness of the gingiva can play an important role in altering soft tissues during orthodontic treatment. There is a high probability of recession during tooth movement in areas with less than 2 mm of gingival thickness [7]. This could affect the integrity of periodontal tissues and represent a risk factor when orthodontic treatments [8], implants [9], and restorative treatments are performed [10]. Gingival biotype is defined as the thickness of the gingiva in the labiolingual direction [9]. Studies have reported that gingival biotype is an important parameter that must be evaluated to reduce the risk of gingival recession [11].

Hence, the assessment of periodontal biotype is considered one of the most important parameters for outcomes focused on dental planning according to the classification of periodontal and peri-implant diseases and conditions [12].

Many features of the gingival phenotype are genetically determined; others seem to be influenced by age, sex, growth, tooth shape, and tooth position [13]. Moreover, it has been shown that among individuals and intra-individual there is variation in the width [14] and thickness of the vestibular gingiva [15].

Facial typology is classified as dolichofacial, mesofacial, or brachyfacial. A dolichofacial typology has excessive vertical facial growth and is usually associated with an increased SellaNasion^GonionGnathion (SN^GoGN) angle and increased vertical jaw relation (AnsPns^GoGn) [16,17]. A brachyfacial typology has reduced vertical growth and is usually accompanied by reduced SN^GoGn, reduced AnsPns^GoGn, and a decreased lower facial height (SNMe) total facial height (NMe) ratio [18].

The cephalometric evaluation of facial type is essential for orthodontic diagnosis because the amount and direction of jaw growth will significantly alter the need for orthodontic biomechanics [19].

Craniofacial morphology may also affect the gingival phenotype [13,20]. Some studies have evaluated the relationship of bone morphology to facial typology [21–23] and a correlation between facial and alveolar bone has already been demonstrated [24]. Indeed, in dolichofacial patients, the mandibular symphysis is high and thin, while in brachyfacial patients, the symphysis is low and thick [25]. As a consequence, before starting orthodontic treatment, it is important to evaluate and to diagnose both the gingival biotype and facial typology with the objective of decreasing the risk of periodontal destruction [26]. Only a few studies have instead evaluated the association between gingival thickness and craniofacial morphology [26].

Facial soft tissue is evaluated using several methodologies; two of the most representative methods, used to obtain three-dimensional (3D) scans, are laser scanners and 3D stereophotogrammetry [27–30]. The analysis of the face using 3D stereophotogrammetry is consistent and valid [31–34]. Hence, this is a reliable method with which to analyze facial soft tissues and avoid any X-ray exposure to the patient [34,35].

Including only patients seeking orthodontic treatment, the aim of this study was to investigate the association between gingival biotype and facial typology evaluated by means of a cephalometric and 3D facial analysis.

The null hypothesis was that there is no association between gingival biotype and facial typology.

2. Materials and Methods

2.1. Subjects

The study sample comprised 121 patients (43 males, 78 females; from 10 to 56 years old, median age 17.04, and interquartile range (IQR) 13.7–22.1) recruited among patients who had to start orthodontic treatment at the Section of Orthodontics and Temporomandibular Disorders of the University of Naples "Federico II".

All patients were fully informed about the nature of the study and signed their informed consent. The research protocol was approved by the Ethics Committee of the University of Naples Federico II (58/19).

The following selection criteria were applied: (1) patients > 8 years, (2) patients had had pre-orthodontic treatment, (3) patients had upper and lower permanent anterior teeth, and (4) patients had good oral hygiene.

Exclusion criteria included diseases requiring premedication to perform periodontal probing, systemic diseases that can influence the activity of periodontal disease, individuals taking drugs that affect periodontal status, patients with removable prostheses, and pregnant or breastfeeding women.

2.2. Periodontal Assessment and Clinical Procedure

Gingival biotype was evaluated based on the transparency of the periodontal probe through the gingival margin of the mid-buccal sulcus of both central and lateral incisors and canines, both maxillary and mandibular. If the outline of the probe could be seen through the gingival margin, it was categorized as "thin" (Figure 1); if not, it was categorized as "thick" (Figure 2) [36].

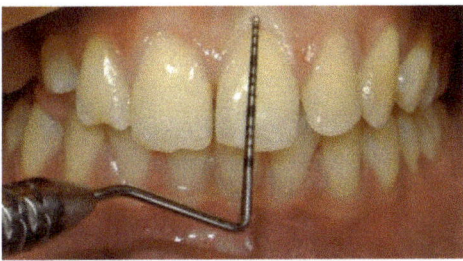

Figure 1. Thin biotype with North Carolina probe.

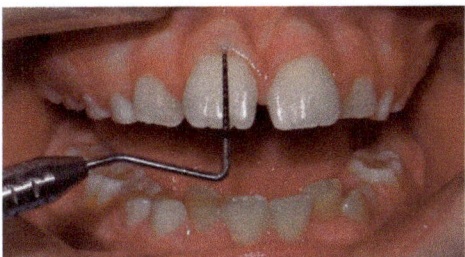

Figure 2. Thick biotype with North Carolina probe.

All the variables were recorded by one expert operator (periodontist) using a millimeter periodontal probe (15 mm North Carolina probe) inserted in the gingival sulcus with a force of about 0.25 Newton.

2.3. D Facial Scans Acquisition Process

The facial scanner 3dMD (3dMD LLC, Atlanta, GA, USA) was used in this study. The scanner was installed in a specific setting, with no lighting (neither natural nor artificial lighting) used during the acquisition.

The scanner configuration consisted of three pairs of stereo-cameras, two texture cameras, and four geometric cameras with lenses slightly convergent, as well as two projectors and three led panels positioned on the right and on the left.

The calibration of the system was the first step of the protocol acquisition. The operator invited the patient to look straight ahead with their head in a natural head position (NHP) for the total scanning time. The teeth were taken together with the eyes opened. After the participant had been properly positioned 90 cm away from the scanner, a video with the six cameras was recorded.

Successively, the scans were exported from the video as .obj images and analyzed using a 3dMDVultus (3dMD LLC, Atlanta, GA, USA). All images were stored on a secure computer in the School of Dentistry at the University of Naples.

2.4. Facial Typology Assessment with Two-Dimensional and Three-Dimensional Cephalometric Evaluation

Delta-Dent software (Outside Format, Spino D'Adda, Italy) was used to perform two-dimensional cephalometric tracings to evaluate facial typology.

For this study, cephalometric analysis was performed as shown in Figure 3a,b. Briefly, two cephalometric variables were assessed: the SNˆGoGn (average value ± SD = 33° ± 2.5°) determined jaw divergence, which is the angle between the anterior cranial base (Sella-Nasion) and the mandibular plane (Gonion-Gnathion), and the CoGoMeˆ angle (average value ± SD = 132° ± 6.0°) that measures the mandibular structure and is formed by the condylar axis (Condylion-Gonion) and the mandibular base (Gonion-Menton).

The sample was divided into three types of craniofacial morphology: brachyfacial, with a SNˆGoGn equal to or lower than 27°, mesofacial, with a SNˆGoGn between 27° and 37°, and dolichofacial, with a SNˆGoGn equal to or greater than 37°.

In order to evaluate facial typology, six points (Figure 3a) were identified and traced on a lateral cephalogram: 'Sella' (S, the center of the sella turcica), 'Nasion' (N, the external point of the junction between the nasal and frontal bones), 'Gonion' (Go, the most inferior posterior point of the mandibular angle), 'Gnathion' (Gn, the point of the mandibular symphysis on the facial axis) 'Menton' (Me, the most inferior point of the mandibular symphysis), and 'Condylion' (Co, the highest and most posterior point on the contour of the mandibular condyle).

The facial scans were acquired and then analyzed using 3dMDVultus Software. On the facial scans, three landmarks were identified: N ('Soft Tissue Nasion', the midpoint on the soft tissue contour of the base of the nasal root at the level of the frontonasal suture), SN ('SubNasion', the midpoint on the nasolabial soft tissue contour between the columella crest and the upper lip), and Me ('Soft Tissue Menton', the most inferior midpoint on the soft tissue contour of the chin). Among these three points, two linear measurements were constructed for the analysis, namely, NMe (total facial height) and SNMe (inferior facial height), as shown in Figure 3c, and the ratio between them was calculated (SNMe/NMe).

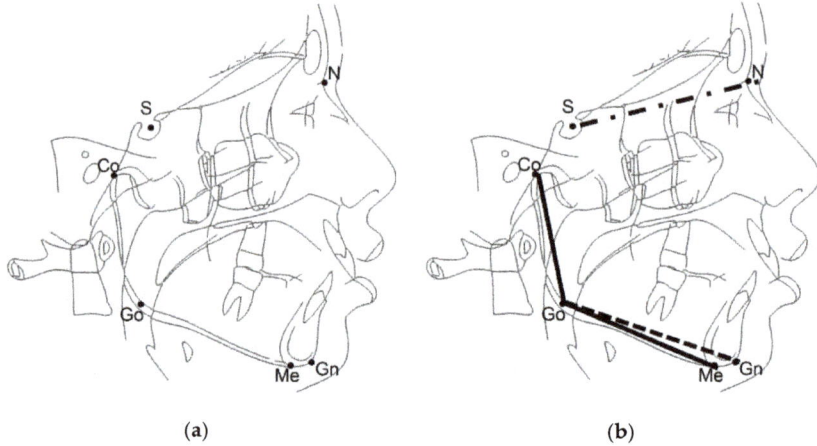

(a) (b)

Figure 3. *Cont.*

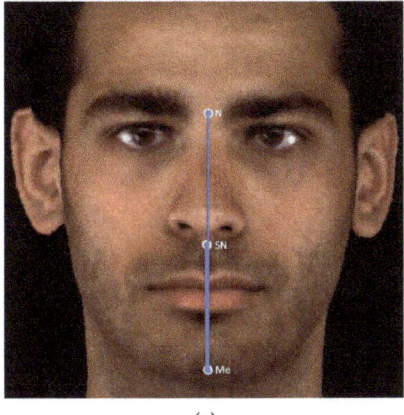

(c)

Figure 3. (a–c) Points, planes, and angles for the assessment of facial typology with cephalometry and facial scanner. (**a**) 'Sellion' (S, the center of the sella turcica), 'Nasion' (N, the external point of the junction between the nasal and frontal bones), 'Gonion' (Go, the most inferior posterior point of the mandibular angle), 'Gnathion' (Gn, the point of the mandibular symphysis on the facial axis) 'Menton' (Me, the most inferior point of the mandibular symphysis), 'Condylion' (Co, the highest and most posterior point on the contour of the mandibular condyle); (**b**) SN plane, GoGn plane, and CoGoMe angle; (**c**) N ('Soft Tissue Nasion', the midpoint on the soft tissue contour of the base of the nasal root at the level of the frontonasal suture), SN ('SubNasion', the midpoint on the nasolabial soft tissue contour between the columella crest and the upper lip), and Me ('Soft Tissue Menton', the most inferior midpoint on the soft tissue contour of the chin). NMe indicates total facial height and SNMe indicates inferior facial height.

2.5. Sample Size

The sample size was established based on the fact that a sample size of 100 patients reaches 80% of power (1-beta) to detect an effect size (W) of 0.31 (medium-large effect size) using a Chi-squared test with two degrees of freedom and a significance level (alpha) of 0.05.

2.6. Statistical Analysis

Descriptive statistics on age, gender, gingival biotype, and baseline characteristics were performed (Table 1). Continuous variables were reported as mean and SD or median and IQR, according to Shapiro-Wilk test, which was performed to evaluate variable distribution. Categorical variables were reported as count and percentage and were compared using the Chi-squared test (gingival biotype versus facial typology). Logistic regression analysis was used to assess the association between continuous variables (CoGoMeˆ and SNMe/NMe) and dichotomous variables (thin or thick biotype) used as dependent variables, including age as a covariate. The level of statistical significance was set at $p < 0.05$. Statistical analysis was performed using STATA version 14.0 (StataCorp. 2015. Stata Statistical Software: Release 14. StataCorp LP: College Station, TX, USA).

3. Results

The total sample consisted of 121 pre-orthodontic patients, comprising 43 males and 78 females which a median age of 17.04 (IQR = 13.7–22.1). Table 1 shows a description of the sample regarding age, sex, gingival biotype, and facial typology. Two-dimensional and 3D cephalometric data are reported in Table 2, and all were normally distributed.

Table 1. Characteristics of study subjects according to age, gender, gingival biotype, and facial typology.

Variables	N	Median (IQR)
Age	121	17.04 (13.7–22.1)
	Frequency	Percentage (%)
Gender		
Male	43	35.54
Female	78	63.64
Upper Gingival Biotype		
Thick	105	86.78
Thin	16	13.22
Lower Gingival Biotype		
Thick	63	52.07
Thin	58	47.93
Facial Typology SNˆGoGn		
Brachyfacial	33	27.27
Mesofacial	59	48.76
Dolichofacial	29	23.97

Data are presented as median and interquartile range (IQR) or frequencies and percentages.

Table 2. Descriptive variables of the sample size.

Variables	Mean ± SD	P50	P25	P75
SNˆGo-Gn	32.7° ± 8°	32.7°	28.1°	36.3°
CoGoMeˆ	123.2° ± 6.6°	122.8°	118.7°	127.4°
SNMe/SMe	0.514 ± 0.042	0.51	0.497	0.530

Data are presented as mean ± SD and IQR. SNˆGoGn (mean ± SD = 33° ± 2.5°) is the angle between the anterior cranial base (Sella-Nasion) and the mandibular plane (Gonion-Gnathion). CoGoMeˆ (average value ± SD = 132° ± 6.0°) is the angle between the condylar axis (Condylion-Gonion) and the mandibular base (Gonion-Menton). SNMe/NMe is the ratio between SNMe (inferior facial height) and NMe (total facial height).

The sample was divided into three groups according to SNˆGoGn, and there were 33 (27.27%) brachyfacial patients, 59 (48.76%) mesofacial patients, and 29 (23.97%) dolichofacial patients, as shown in Table 1.

Regarding gingival biotype, most patients presented a thick gingival biotype (upper anterior teeth (UGB) 86.78%; lower anterior teeth (LGB) 52.07%), as seen in Table 1.

The Chi-squared test showed that there was no statistically significant association between SNˆGoGn and gingival biotype (UGB $p = 0.83$; LGB $p = 0.75$; and gingival biotype $p = 0.77$, Table 3).

Similarly, the logistic regression analysis showed that CoGoMeˆ was not associated with any variables of gingival biotype (UGB, $p = 0.340$; LGB, $p = 0.065$).

Finally, logistic regression analysis showed a statistically significant association of SNMe/NMe with the UGB (odds ratio = 0.843; 95% CI 0.719–0.989; $p = 0.036$) and of SNMe/NMe with LGB (odds ratio = 0.904; 95% CI 0.818–1.000; $p = 0.049$), showing that when the ratio of SNMe/NMe decreases, there is a minor risk of finding a thin biotype (Table 4).

Table 3. Classification of gingival biotype in patients with different facial typologies (classified according to SNˆGoGn) using a 15 mm North Carolina probe.

Facial Typology (N)	Upper Gingival Biotype		
	Thick	Thin	p value
Brachyfacial (33)	29 (27.62%)	4 (25.00%)	0.83
Mesofacial (59)	50 (47.62%)	9 (56.25%)	
Dolichofacial (29)	26 (24.76%)	3 (18.75%)	
Total (121)	105 (100%)	16 (100%)	
	Lower Gingival Biotype		
	Thick	Thin	p value
Brachyfacial (33)	16 (25.40%)	17 (29.31%)	0.75
Mesofacial (59)	33 (52.38%)	26 (44.83%)	
Dolichofacial (29)	14 (22.22%)	15 (25.86%)	
Total (121)	63 (100%)	58 (100%)	
	Gingival Biotype			
	Thick/Thick	Thick/Thin	Thin/Thin	p value
Brachyfacial (33)	16 (25.40%)	13 (30.95%)	4 (25%)	0.77
Mesofacial (59)	33 (52.38%)	17 (40.48%)	9 (56.25%)	
Dolichofacial (29)	14 (22.22%)	12 (28.57%)	3 (18.75%)	
Total (121)	63 (100%)	42 (100%)	16 (100%)	

Data are presented as numbers, percentages, and p values.

Table 4. Logistic regression model for SNMe/NMe ratio × 100 with and without including age as a coviariate.

Model	Variable	p Value	Odds Ratio (OR)	95% IC
Upper biotype (SNMe/NMe)	SNMe/NMe	0.036 *	0.843	0.719–0.989
Lower biotype (SNMe/NMe)	SNMe/NMe	0.049 *	0.904	0.818–0.999
Upper biotype (SNMe/NMe × Age)	SNMe/NMe	0.034 *	0.839	0.714–0.987
	Age	0.620	0.985	0.927–1.046
Lower biotype (SNMe/NMe × Age)	SNMe/NMe	0.048 *	0.903	0.815–0.999
	Age	0.207	0.976	0.939–1.014

Data are presented as OR and IQR. * and bold text indicate statistically significant values ($p < 0.05$).

4. Discussion

The aim of this study was to investigate the association between facial typology and gingival biotype in pre-orthodontic patients in order to guarantee a better diagnosis and planning of orthodontic treatment.

We tested whether the facial typology measured on two-dimensional cephalograms (SNˆGoGn and CoGoMeˆ) or on three-dimensional facial scans (SNMe/NMe) could affect gingival biotype. No association was found between facial typology assessed using the two-dimensional angles SNˆGoGn or CoGoMeˆ and maxillary and mandibular gingival biotype of the anterior regions. There is one study that correlates craniofacial morphology using magnetic resonance imaging (MRI) with tooth root exposure and periodontal attachment loss. The study used the ratio of facial width and length (facial index) to describe craniofacial morphology and showed that patients with long narrow faces were associated with higher loss of attachment [37].

A recent study performed by Kaya et al. has investigated the relationship between gingival phenotype and craniofacial morphology in the sagittal and vertical directions. In contrast to this research, an endodontic file, namely, transgingival probing, was used to assess gingival phenotype (<1 mm and >1 mm, thin and thick phenotype, respectively). These results demonstrated that there is no association between gingival thickness and craniofacial typology [26].

In this study, facial typology was also evaluated with three-dimensional facial scans to assess the association between SNMe/NMe and gingival thickness. Our analysis showed that facial proportions have a statistically significant association with gingival biotype. In particular, when the ratio of SNMe/NMe is decreased, there is a minor risk of finding a thin gingival biotype either in the upper or lower anterior regions.

This is the first study that has evaluated gingival thickness through the periodontal probe's translucency (thin and adequate biotype) with different vertical facial heights, and these findings support the hypothesis that there is no correlation between facial morphology and gingival thickness on lateral cephalograms [24]. Gingival thickness can be assessed by transgingival probing [38], ultrasonic measurement [39], or through the visibility of the probe [40,41]. Transgingival probing was not used because of the need for local anesthesia, which could induce a local volume increase and discomfort for patients [38]. Additionally, ultrasonic measurement was not preferred because of its repeatability with a coefficient of 1.20 mm [42]. Instead, the transparency of the probe through the gingival margin has been found to have a high reproducibility by De Rouck et al., showing 85% inter-examiner repeatability (k value = 0.7, p value = 0.002) [40]. Thus, this study used the periodontal probe visible through the gingiva after its placement in the facial sulcus of the anterior teeth [40].

The prevalence of malocclusion can vary between children and adolescents. However, the demand for orthodontic treatment is increasing [43–45], and greater attention has to be paid to periodontal aspects; indeed, orthodontic treatment can play an important role in periodontal changes [46]. The thickness of the gingiva is supposed to represent an indicator for reducing the risk of bone loss and gingival recession [47]. In fact, there are two studies which have indicated a statistically significant relationship between facial biotype and alveolar height and thickness with a greater risk of moving incisors beyond the anatomic limits of the alveolar bone by application of uncontrolled forces [6,48]. This uncontrolled movement can bring to: alveolar bone fenestrations, increasing susceptibility to gingival recession [49,50] and recession in the case of less than 2 mm of gingival thickness [7].

The current study presents several strengths. First, the periodontal assessments were performed in all of patients at the beginning of orthodontic treatment. This allows for an accurate diagnosis and treatment planning. In order to avoid bias due to differences in operator performance, only two trained clinicians performed the periodontal evaluations. Moreover, a new method to evaluate craniofacial morphology was introduced without exposure to the patients of further radiation. The study also has some limitations. Firstly, the sample size was relatively small to achieve a more reliable result. Secondly, only a few patients presented a thin UGB; however, this was in accordance with the normal prevalence of this biotype [26]. Further longitudinal studies are necessary to monitor the long-term effects of orthodontic treatment on gingival biotype in different facial typologies.

5. Conclusions

1. There is no association between facial typology (evaluated with SN^GoGn and CoGoMe) and gingival biotype.
2. When the ratio of SNMe/NMe is decreased, it represents a protective factor and a minor risk of finding a thin gingival biotype.

Author Contributions: Conceptualization, V.D., R.R. and R.V.; Methodology, A.P., R.R., V.S. and V.D.; Validation, A.P., G.S., G.T., and R.V.; Formal Analysis, A.P., G.T., R.R., and V.S.; Investigation, A.P., G.T. and R.R.; Resources, V.D. and R.V.; Data Curation, A.P., G.T., R.R. and V.S.; Writing–Original Draft Preparation, A.P., R.R. and V.D.; Writing–Review & Editing, G.T., V.S., G.S. and R.V.; Visualization, A.P., G.T., and R.R.; Supervision, G.S., V.D. and R.V.; Project Administration, A.P., V.D. and R.R.

Funding: This research received no external funding.

Conflicts of Interest: The authors declare no conflict of interest.

References

1. Liu, P.; Liu, Y.; Wang, J.; Guo, Y.; Zhang, Y.; Xiao, S. Detection of fusobacterium nucleatum and fada adhesin gene in patients with orthodontic gingivitis and non-orthodontic periodontal inflammation. *PLoS ONE* **2014**, *9*, e85280. [CrossRef] [PubMed]
2. Bollen, A.; Cunha-cruz, J.; Bakko, W.; Huang, G.J.; Hujoel, P.P. The Effects of Orthodontic Therapy on Periodontal Health: A Systematic Review of Controlled Evidence. *J. Am. Dent. Assoc.* **2008**, *139*, 413–422. [CrossRef] [PubMed]
3. Tanner, A.C.R.; Sonis, A.L.; Lif Holgerson, P.; Starr, J.R.; Nunez, Y.; Kressirer, C.A.; Paster, B.J.; Johansson, I. White-spot lesions and gingivitis microbiotas in orthodontic patients. *J. Dent. Res.* **2012**, *91*, 853–858. [CrossRef] [PubMed]
4. Renkema, A.M.; Navratilova, Z.; Mazurova, K.; Katsaros, C.; Fudalej, P.S. Gingival labial recessions and the post-treatment proclination of mandibular incisors. *Eur. J. Orthod.* **2015**, *37*, 508–513. [CrossRef]
5. Renkema, A.M.; Fudalej, P.S.; Renkema, A.A.P.; Abbas, F.; Bronkhorst, E.; Katsaros, C. Gingival labial recessions in orthodontically treated and untreated individuals: A case-Control study. *J. Clin. Periodontol.* **2013**, *40*, 631–637. [CrossRef]
6. Morris, J.W.; Campbell, P.M.; Tadlock, L.P.; Boley, J.; Buschang, P.H. Prevalence of gingival recession after orthodontic tooth movements. *Am. J. Orthod. Dentofac. Orthop.* **2017**, *151*, 851–859. [CrossRef]
7. Kim, D.M.; Neiva, R. Periodontal Soft Tissue Non–Root Coverage Procedures: A Systematic Review From the AAP Regeneration Workshop. *J. Periodontol.* **2015**, *86*, S56–S72. [CrossRef]
8. Joss-Vassalli, I.; Grebenstein, C.; Topouzelis, N.; Sculean, A.; Katsaros, C. Orthodontic therapy and gingival recession: A systematic review. *Orthod. C. Res.* **2010**, *13*, 127–141. [CrossRef]
9. Kois, J.C. Predictable single-tooth peri-implant esthetics: Five diagnostic keys. *Compend. Contin. Educ. Dent.* **2004**, *25*, 895–896.
10. Ahmad, I. Anterior dental aesthetics: Gingival perspective. *Br. Dent. J.* **2005**, *199*, 195–202. [CrossRef]
11. Grover, V.; Bhardwaj, A.; Mohindra, K.; Malhotra, R. Analysis of the gingival biotype based on the measurement of the dentopapillary complex. *J. Indian Soc. Periodontol.* **2014**, *18*, 43. [CrossRef] [PubMed]
12. Papapanou, P.N.; Sanz, M.; Buduneli, N.; Dietrich, T.; Feres, M.; Fine, D.H.; Flemmig, T.F.; Garcia, R.; Giannobile, W.V.; Graziani, F.; et al. Periodontitis: Consensus report of workgroup 2 of the 2017 World Workshop on the Classification of Periodontal and Peri-Implant Diseases and Conditions. *J. Clin. Periodontol.* **2018**, *89*, S173–S182. [CrossRef] [PubMed]
13. Vandana, K.L.; Savitha, B. Thickness of gingiva in association with age, gender and dental arch location. *J. Clin. Periodontol.* **2005**, *32*, 828–830. [CrossRef] [PubMed]
14. Seibert, J.; Lindhe, J. Aestetics and periodontal therapy. In *Textbook of Clinical Periodontology*, 2nd ed.; Munksgaard: Copenhagen, Denmark, 1989; pp. 477–514.
15. Olsson, M.; Lindhe, J. Periodontal characteristics in individuals with varying form of the upper central incisors. *J. Clin. Periodontol.* **1991**, *18*, 78–82. [CrossRef]
16. Fields, H.; Proffit, W.; Nixon, W.; Phillips, C.; Stanek, E. Facial pattern differences in long-faced children and adults. *Am. J. Orthod.* **1984**, *85*, 217–223. [CrossRef]
17. Cangialosi, T.J. Additional criteria for sample division suggested. *Am. J. Orthod. Dentofac. Orthop.* **1989**, *96*, A24. [CrossRef]
18. Opdebeeck, H.; Bell, W. The short face syndrome. *Am. J. Orthod.* **1978**, *73*, 499–511. [CrossRef]
19. Schudy, F.F. The Rotation of The Mandible Resulting From Growth: Its Implications In Orthodontic Treatment. *Angle Orthod.* **1964**, *34*, 75–93.
20. Matarese, G.; Isola, G.; Ramaglia, L.; Dalessandri, D.; Lucchese, A.; Alibrandi, A.; Fabiano, F.; Cordasco, G. Periodontal biotype: Characteristc, prevalence and dimension related to dental malocclusion. *Minerva Stomatol.* **2016**, *65*, 231–238.
21. Al-Zo'ubia, I.A.; Hammadb, M.M.; Abu Alhaijac, E.S.J. Periodontal parameters in different dentofacial vertical patterns. *Angle Orthod.* **2008**, *78*, 1006–1014. [CrossRef]
22. Hornera, K.A.; Behrents, R.G.; Beom Kim, K.; Buschangd, P.H. Cortical bone and ridge thickness of hyperdivergent and hypodivergent adults. *Am. J. Orthod. Dentofac. Orthop.* **2012**, *142*, 170–178. [CrossRef] [PubMed]

23. Esfahanizadeh, N.; Daneshparvar, N.; Askarpour, F.; Akhoundi, N.; Panjnoush, M. Correlation Between Bone and Soft Tissue Thickness in Maxillary Anterior Teeth. *J. Dent. (Tehran)* **2016**, *13*, 302–308.
24. Sadek, M.M.; Sabet, N.E.; Hassan, I.T. Alveolar bone mapping in subjects with different vertical facial dimensions. *Eur. J. Orthod.* **2014**, *37*, 194–201. [CrossRef] [PubMed]
25. Björk, A. Prediction of mandibular growth rotation. *Am. J. Orthod.* **1969**, *55*, 585–599. [CrossRef]
26. Kaya, Y.; Alkan, Ö.; Alkan, E.A.; Keskin, S. Gingival thicknesses of maxillary and mandibular anterior regions in subjects with different craniofacial morphologies. *Am. J. Orthod. Dentofac. Orthop.* **2018**, *154*, 356–364. [CrossRef] [PubMed]
27. Baik, H.S.; Kim, S.Y. Facial soft-tissue changes in skeletal Class III orthognathic surgery patients analyzed with 3-dimensional laser scanning. *Am. J. Orthod. Dentofac. Orthop.* **2010**, *138*, 167–178. [CrossRef] [PubMed]
28. Kau, C.H.; Richmond, S.; Incrapera, A.; English, J.; Xia, J.J. Three-dimensional surface acquisition systems for the study of facial morphology and their application to maxillofacial surgery. *Int. J. Med. Robot. Comput. Assist. Surg.* **2007**, *3*, 97–110. [CrossRef]
29. Staderini, E.; Patini, R.; De Luca, M.; Gallenzi, P. Three-dimensional stereophotogrammetric analysis of nasolabial soft tissue effects of rapid maxillary expansion: A systematic review of clinical trials. *Acta Otorhinolaryngol. Ital.* **2018**, *38*, 399–408.
30. Antoun, J.S.; Lawrence, C.; Leow, A.; Rongo, R.; Dias, G.; Farella, M. A three-dimensional evaluation of Māori and New Zealand European faces. *Aust. Orthod. J.* **2014**, *30*, 169.
31. Aynechi, N.; Larson, B.E.; Leon-Salazar, V.; Beiraghi, S. Accuracy and precision of a 3D anthropometric facial analysis with and without landmark labeling before image acquisition. *Angle Orthod.* **2011**, *81*, 245–252. [CrossRef]
32. Plooij, J.M.; Swennen, G.R.J.; Rangel, F.A.; Maal, T.J.J.; Schutyser, F.A.C.; Bronkhorst, E.M.; Kuijpers-Jagtman, A.M.; Bergé, S.J. Evaluation of reproducibility and reliability of 3D soft tissue analysis using 3D stereophotogrammetry. *Int. J. Oral Maxillofac. Surg.* **2009**, *38*, 267–273. [CrossRef] [PubMed]
33. Toma, A.M.; Zhurov, A.; Playle, R.; Ong, E.; Richmond, S. Reproducibility of facial soft tissue landmarks on 3D laser-scanned facial images. *Orthod. Craniofac. Res.* **2009**, *12*, 33–42. [CrossRef] [PubMed]
34. Rongo, R.; Antoun, J.S.; Lim, Y.X.; Dias, G.; Valletta, R.; Farella, M. Three-dimensional evaluation of the relationship between jaw divergence and facial soft tissue dimensions. *Angle Orthod.* **2014**, *84*, 788–794. [CrossRef] [PubMed]
35. Young, N.M.; Sherathiya, K.; Gutierrez, L.; Nguyen, E.; Bekmezian, S.; Huang, J.C.; Hallgrimsson, B.; Lee, J.S.; Marcucio, R.S. Facial surface morphology predicts variation in internal skeletal shape. *Am. J. Orthod. Dentofac. Orthop.* **2016**, *149*, 501–508. [CrossRef]
36. Kan, J.Y.K.; Rungcharassaeng, K.; Umezu, K.; Kois, J.C. Dimensions of Peri-Implant Mucosa: An Evaluation of Maxillary Anterior Single Implants in Humans. *J. Periodontol.* **2003**, *74*, 557–562. [CrossRef]
37. Salti, L.; Holtfreter, B.; Pink, C.; Habes, M.; Biffar, R.; Kiliaridis, S.; Krey, K.F.; Bülow, R.; Völzke, H.; Kocher, T.; et al. Estimating effects of craniofacial morphology on gingival recession and clinical attachment loss. *J. Clin. Periodontol.* **2017**, *44*, 363–371. [CrossRef]
38. Ronay, V.; Sahrmann, P.; Bindl, A.; Attin, T.; Schmidlin, P.R. Current status and perspectives of mucogingival soft tissue measurement methods. *J. Esthet. Restor. Dent.* **2011**, *23*, 146–156. [CrossRef]
39. Eger, T.; Muller, H.-P.; Heinecke, A. Ultrasonic determination of gingival thickness subject variation and influence of tooth type and clinical features. *J. Clin. Periodontol.* **1996**, *23*, 839–845. [CrossRef]
40. De Rouck, T.; Eghbali, R.; Collys, K.; De Bruyn, H.; Cosyn, J. The gingival biotype revisited: Transparency of the periodontal probe through the gingival margin as a method to discriminate thin from thick gingiva. *J. Clin. Periodontol.* **2009**, *36*, 428–433. [CrossRef]
41. Cortellini, P.; Bissada, N.F. Mucogingival conditions in the natural dentition: Narrative review, case definitions, and diagnostic considerations. *J. Clin. Periodontol.* **2018**, *45*, S190–S198. [CrossRef]
42. Müller, H.P.; Könönen, E. Variance components of gingival thickness. *J. Periodontal Res.* **2005**, *40*, 239–244. [CrossRef] [PubMed]
43. Paduano, S.; Rongo, R.; Bucci, R.; Aiello, D.; Carvelli, G.; Ingenito, A.; Cantile, T.; Ferrazzano, G.F. Is there an association between various aspects of oral health in Southern Italy children? An epidemiological study assessing dental decays, periodontal status, malocclusions and temporomandibular joint function. *Eur. J. Paediatr. Dent.* **2018**, *19*, 176–180. [PubMed]

44. Asiri, S.N.; Tadlock, L.P.; Buschang, P.H. The prevalence of clinically meaningful malocclusion among US adults. *Orthod. Craniofac. Res.* **2019**, *22*, 321–328. [CrossRef]
45. Jawad, Z.; Bates, C.; Hodge, T. Who needs orthodontic treatment? Who gets it? And who wants it? *Br. Dent. J.* **2015**, *218*, 99–103. [CrossRef]
46. Alfuriji, S.; Alhazmi, N.; Alhamlan, N.; Al-Ehaideb, A.; Alruwaithi, M.; Alkatheeri, N.; Geevarghese, A. The effect of orthodontic therapy on periodontal health: A review of the literature. *Int. J. Dent.* **2014**, *2014*, 585048. [CrossRef]
47. Maynard, J.G. The rationale for mucogingival therapy in the child and adolescent. *Int. J. Periodontics Restor. Dent.* **1987**, *7*, 36–51.
48. Renkema, A.M.; Fudalej, P.S.; Renkema, A.; Kiekens, R.; Katsaros, C. Development of labial gingival recessions in orthodontically treated patients. *Am. J. Orthod. Dentofac. Orthop.* **2013**, *143*, 206–212. [CrossRef]
49. Holmesa, H.D.; Tennantb, M.; Goonewardenec, M.S. Augmentation of faciolingual gingival dimensions with free connective tissue grafts before labial orthodontic tooth movement: An experimental study with a canine model. *Am. J. Orthod. Dentofac. Orthop.* **2005**, *127*, 562–572. [CrossRef]
50. Wennström, J.L.; Lindhe, J.; Sinclair, F.; Thilander, B. Some periodontal tissue reactions to orthodontic tooth movement in monkeys. *J. Clin. Periodontol.* **1987**, *14*, 121–129. [CrossRef]

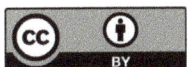 © 2019 by the authors. Licensee MDPI, Basel, Switzerland. This article is an open access article distributed under the terms and conditions of the Creative Commons Attribution (CC BY) license (http://creativecommons.org/licenses/by/4.0/).

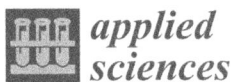

Review

Surface Alterations Induced on Endodontic Instruments by Sterilization Processes, Analyzed with Atomic Force Microscopy: A Systematic Review

Mario Dioguardi [1,*], Vito Crincoli [2], Luigi Laino [3], Mario Alovisi [4], Enrica Laneve [1], Diego Sovereto [1], Bruna Raddato [1], Khrystyna Zhurakivska [1], Filiberto Mastrangelo [1], Domenico Ciavarella [1], Lucio Lo Russo [1] and Lorenzo Lo Muzio [1]

1. Department of Clinical and Experimental Medicine, University of Foggia, Via Rovelli 50, 71122 Foggia, Italy; enrica.laneve@unifg.it (E.L.); diego_sovereto.546709@unifg.it (D.S.); brunaraddato@gmail.com (B.R.); khrystyna.zhurakivska@unifg.it (K.Z.); filiberto.mastrangelo@unifg.it (F.M.); domenico.ciavarella@unifg.it (D.C.); lucio.lorusso@unifg.it (L.L.R.); lorenzo.lomuzio@unifg.it (L.L.M.)
2. Department of Basic Medical Sciences, Neurosciences and Sensory Organs, Division of Complex Operating Unit of Dentistry, "Aldo Moro" University of Bari, Piazza G. Cesare 11, 70124 Bari, Italy; vito.crincoli@uniba.it
3. Multidisciplinary Department of Medical-Surgical and Odontostomatological Specialties, University of Campania "Luigi Vanvitelli", 80121 Naples, Italy; luigi.laino@unicampania.it
4. Department of Surgical Sciences, Dental School, University of Turin, 10124 Turin, Italy; mario.alovisi@unito.it
* Correspondence: mario.dioguardi@unifg.it

Received: 29 October 2019; Accepted: 14 November 2019; Published: 17 November 2019

Abstract: Endodontic canal disinfection procedures that use sodium hypochlorite, and subsequently, heat sterilization procedures can alter the surface of endodontic instruments, described as corrosion and micropitting. These phenomena can be visualized on the surface of the instruments by SEM and atomic force microscopy analyses. The endodontic instruments used in probing, pre-enlargement, and shaping phases are made of steel alloy or nickel-titanium alloy (NiTi) and are subject to torsional, flexor, and cyclic fatigue; indeed, reuse of these instruments must be done with the knowledge that these instruments are subject to fracture following stress caused during their use. Fracture of the instrument within the canal is an eventuality that can lead to failure of the treatment, and therefore it is important to try to reduce situations that can contribute to the fracture. This review was performed based on the PRISMA protocol. Studies were identified through bibliographic research using electronic databases. A total of 1036 records were identified on the PubMed and Scopus databases. After screening the articles, restricted by year of publication (1979 to 2019), there were 946 records. With the application of the eligibility criteria (all the articles pertaining to the issue of sterilization in endodontics), there were 228 articles. There were 104 articles after eliminating overlaps. There were 50 articles that discussed the influence of sterilization procedures on the surface characteristics of endodontic instruments, and 26 articles that measured parameters on surface alteration. Applying the inclusion and exclusion criteria resulted in a total of eleven articles for quantitative analysis. Four articles were in reference to the primary outcome, eight articles to secondary outcome, and five articles to tertiary outcome. The meta-analysis showed a statistically significant surface alteration effect after five autoclaves and after immersion in the canal irrigants after 10 min.

Keywords: autoclave; endodontic sterilization; atomic force microscopy; NiTi alloy; endodontics; corrosion

1. Introduction

Endodontic instruments are commonly used in dental practice to perform endodontic treatments of vital and necrotic teeth, endodontic retreatments, pulpotomies, pulpectomy and specification procedures. Depending on the phase of treatment, endodontic instruments are divided into instruments for probing the endodontic canal for the pre-enlargement, and glidepath for shaping the canal or instruments for the closure and three-dimensional sealing of endodontic canals [1,2]. Many of these tools are reusable after performing cleaning, disinfection, and sterilization procedures by autoclaving [3].

Endodontic canal disinfection procedures that use sodium hypochlorite [4], and subsequently, heat sterilization procedures, can alter the surface of endodontic instruments, described as corrosion and micropitting, phenomena [5] that can be visualized by SEM and atomic force microscopy analyses.

The endodontic instruments used in the probing, pre-enlargement, and shaping phases are made of steel alloy or nickel-titanium alloy (NiTi) and are subject to torsional, flexor, and cyclic fatigue, indeed the reuse of these instruments must be done with the knowledge that these tools are subject to fracture following stress caused during their use [6]. Fracture of the instrument within the canal is an eventuality that can lead to failure of the treatment, and therefore it is important to try to reduce situations that can contribute the fracture.

On the surface subject to fatigue, surface alterations can give rise to microcrack which can lead to fracture of the instrument, and also reduce the cutting capacity of the blades on the endodontic files [7]. Therefore, in order to maintain the same cutting efficiency, the endodontist has to exert greater pressure on the instrument with an increase in torsional fatigue stress [6].

An atomic force microscope is an instrument capable of analyzing the surface of instruments. It consists of a cantilever with a pointed tip (tip) mounted on the end, typically composed of silicon or silicon nitride and having a radius of curvature of the "order of nanometers". The sample to be scanned, through the Vand Der Waals forces, interacts with the tip of the detector by flexing it. There are several methods to detect any cantilever movement. The majority of atomic force microscopy (AFM) systems use laser beam detection, which is an optical system with position sensitive detectors called photodiodes. The laser light is reflected by the cantilever on the position-sensitive photodiode. Very small forces are produced between the probe and the surface to be scanned, and these are the forces that allow the AFM system to record the deflection of the cantilever. The cantilever deflection is called "cantilever rigidity". This rigidity can be measured by Hooke's law. Rigidity is recorded visually and can be viewed on the computer in real time. The surface scan of endodontic instruments is used both in non-contact mode and in contact mode and, in general, the scanned surfaces start at 3 mm from the tip of the instrument up to 6 mm. The parameters which are considered with AFM for the analysis of a surface are the arithmetic mean roughness(AMR) of the maximum height (MH) and root mean square (RMS). The atomic force microscopy, therefore, provides detailed information with measurable parameters of possible alterations and irregularities present on the surface of an instrument [8].

Surface alterations can represent a problem in the use of endodontic instruments. A study by Ylmaz, in 2018, identified surface alterations described as surface roughness with statistically significant results for instruments constructed with new M-wire and EDM alloys [9].

One problem of reusing endodontic instruments that are subject to fatigue is the deterioration they suffer that results from their use in the dental canal for the removal of dentin, as well as the corrosive action by the root canal irrigants such as sodium hypochlorite, and subsequently, the action of the temperature and steam induced by the autoclave sterilization process. The surface alterations are well described in a study by Inan, in 2007, on the universal ProTaper, after clinical use and sterilization [10].

Fayyad and Mahran, in a 2013 study, demonstrated by AFM analysis that the alterations on Twisted Files [11], Hero Shaper, RaCe, and GTX instruments were statistically significant after immersion in 5% sodium hypochlorite, however, the alterations were not statistically significant after EDTA immersion. In contrast, Ametrano et al., in 2010, reported significant results for instruments immersed in EDTA [12]. Other studies have report conflicting data, such as the study conducted by Casella, in 2011, in which there was no variation in corrosion resistance for some instruments (K FILE and GT-rotary) unlike the K3 knife immersed in 5% sodium hypochlorite [13]. In addition, studies conducted at the Sem da Razavianet, in 2015, reported an increase in roughness directly related to the number of sterilization cycles performed on endodontic instruments [14].

In contrast, there is debate within the scientific community regarding whether there are statistically significant surface alterations induced by the autoclave or the canal irrigants. This review aims to try to clarify this aspect by investigating the literature to extrapolate the data on surface alterations in endodontic instruments in order to statistically analyze them in a meta-analysis.

Previous systematic reviews on this topic have not included the effect of surface alterations of endodontic instruments subjected to heat sterilization. There is only one systematic review that analyzes the variations in torsional properties subjected to autoclave sterilization.

This review could help endodontists who perform endodontic therapy and reuse endodontic instruments daily. Awareness of the greater or lesser risk of potential fracture triggered by surface variations due to heat or use of canal irrigants on the instruments could be helpful.

2. Materials and Methods

This systematic review was conducted based on the Prisma protocol.

The study was constructed using the following PICO elements for questions: Population (endodontic instruments); intervention (surface alterations induced by sterilization processes and root canal irrigation); control (new endodontic instruments not subject to sterilization; and outcome (surface alterations induced by the sterilization process by autoclave, and by root canal irrigants such as sodium hypochlorite and EDTA).

The following PICO question was formulated: To what extent, statistically significant, the sterilization processes and the used canal irrigants alter the surface of the rotating endodontic instruments with respect to the control?

After an initial selection phase of article identification in the databases, the potentially eligible articles were qualitatively evaluated in order to investigate the surface alterations of endodontic instruments resulting from the sterilization of instruments and disinfection of endodontic canals.

2.1. Eligibility Criteria

This literature review took into consideration in vitro and clinical studies that concerned the subject of sterilization and the influence of the latter on the physical and chemical properties of endodontic instruments. In particular, articles that dealt with the corrosive phenomena and surface alterations considered by microscopy methods (atomic force microscopy), conducted in recent years, and published with abstracts in English, were considered potentially eligible.

Articles from the last 40 years were chosen, because disinfection and sterilization procedures have changed in light of new discovered infectious contaminants, such as HIV and HCV viruses and the prong of spongiform encephalopathy. Furthermore, the methods used to manufacture the instruments have changed with the introduction of new alloys and new instruments. Therefore, in summary, potentially eligible articles included studies that investigated the influence of sterilization and disinfection procedures on endodontic canals, as well as on the physical and chemical characteristics of endodontic instruments, however, articles published more than 40 years ago and those that did not present an abstract in English were excluded.

Finally, the articles that were potentially eligible were subjected to a full text analysis to verify their use for a qualitative and quantitative analysis.

The inclusion and exclusion criteria applied in the full text analysis are the following:

- Include all those studies that describe the alterations induced by the sterilization methods of the endodontic instruments, analyzed using atomic force microscopy;
- Include all the articles that describe the alterations induced by root canal irrigants (sodium hypochlorite and EDTA), analyzed using atomic force microscopy;
- The exclusion criteria are to exclude all those studies that do not report data (average and standard deviation) on surface irregularities (AMR, MH, and RMS).

2.2. Research Methodology

The studies were identified through a bibliographic research on electronic databases.

The literature search was conducted using the search engines "PubMed" and "Scopus". The search on the providers was conducted between 12 September 2019 and 18 September 2019 and the last search for a partial update of the literature was conducted on 1 October 2019.

The following search terms were used on PubMed and Scopus: "Endodontic sterilization" PubMed 333 and Scopus 269; "endodontic autoclave" PubMed 38 and Scopus 52; "atomic force microscopy" AND "endodontic" PubMed 21 and Scopus 33; "roughness" AND "endodontic" Pub Med 42 and Scopus 67; "roughness" AND "ethylenediaminetetraacetic acid" PubMed 15 and Scopus 40; "roughness" AND "sodium hypochlorite" PubMed 1 and Scopus 1; "sodium hypochlorite" AND "atomic force microscopy" PubMed 40 and Scopus 80; "atomic force microscopy" AND "NiTi rotary instruments" PubMed 1 and Scopus 2 (Table 1).

2.3. Screening Methodology

The records obtained were, subsequently, examined by two independent reviewers (M.D. and S.D), and a third reviewer (E.L.) acted as a decision maker in situations of doubt. The screening included the analysis of the title and the abstract to eliminate the recordings not related to the topics of the review. After the screening phase, the overlaps were removed and the complete texts of the articles were analyzed, from which the ones eligible for the qualitative analysis and the inclusion in the meta-analysis for the three results were identified. The results sought by the two reviewers were:

(1) Primary outcome, variations of the root mean square root (RMS) of endodontic instruments subjected to five autoclave cycles as compared with non-autoclaved control;
(2) Secondary outcome, variations of the root mean square (RMS) of endodontic instruments exposed to sodium hypochlorite 5% as compared with the control group;
(3) Tertiary outcome, variations of the root mean square (RMS) of the endodontic instruments described at EDTA 10% as compared with the control group.

The fourth reviewer, with supervisory duties, was L.Lo.M. The K agreement between the two screening reviewers was 0.8464 (Table 2). The K agreement was based on the formulas of the *Cochrane Handbook for Systematic Reviews* [15].

The Newcastle–Ottawa scale for case-control studies was used to assess the risk of bias in the included studies. The quantitative analysis was performed with the Rev Manager software 5.3 (Cochrane Collaboration, Copenhagen, Denmark [16].

Table 1. Complete overview of the search methodology.

Database-Provider	Key Words	Search Details	Number of Records	Number of Records after Restriction by Year of Publication (Last 40 Years)	Number of Articles Remaining after the Elimination of Records not Related to the Issue of Sterilization Influence on Endodontic Instruments	Articles After Remove Overlaps Articles	Number of Articles Dealing with the Problem of the Influence of Sterilization Procedures on the Surface Characteristics of Endodontic Instruments	Number of Articles that Have Analyzed the Surface Alterations with Methods Different from the Atomic Force Microscopy	Number of Articles that Analyzed Surface Alterations with Atomic Force Microscopy	Numbers of Articles Included in the Quantitative Analysis for the 3 Outcomes
PubMed	"endodontic sterilization"	"endodontic" [All Fields] AND ("sterilization" [All Fields] OR "sterilization", reproductive" [MeSH Terms] OR ("sterilization" [All Fields] AND "reproductive" [All Fields]) OR "reproductive sterilization" [All Fields] OR "sterilization" [MeSH Terms])	333	291	46					
PubMed	"endodontic autoclave"	"endodontic" [All Fields] AND "autoclave" [All Fields]	38	38	25					
PubMed	"atomic force microscopy" AND "endodontic"	"atomic force microscopy" [All Fields] AND "endodontic" [All Fields]	21	21	9					
PubMed	"roughness" AND "endodontic"	"roughness" [All Fields] AND "endodontic" [All Fields]	42	41	11					
PubMed	"roughness" AND "ethylenediaminetetraacetic acid"	"roughness" [All Fields] AND ("ethylenediaminetetraacetic" [All Fields] AND "acid" [All Fields])	15	15	2					
PubMed	"roughness" AND "sodium hypochlorite"	"roughness" [All Fields] AND ("sodium" [All Fields] AND "hypochlorite" [All Fields])	1	1	1					
PubMed	"sodium" "hypochlorite" AND "atomic force microscopy"	"sodium hypochlorite" [All Fields] AND "atomic force microscopy" [All Fields]	40	40	13					
PubMed	"atomic force microscopy" AND "NiTi rotary instruments"	"atomic force microscopy" [All Fields] AND "NiTi rotary instruments" [All Fields]	1	1	1					
Scopus	"endodontic sterilization"	TITLE-ABS-KEY (endodontic AND sterilization)	269	225	56					
Scopus	"endodontic autoclave"	TITLE-ABS-KEY (endodontic AND autoclave)	52	52	25					
Scopus	"atomic force microscopy" AND "endodontic"	TITLE-ABS-KEY ("atomic force microscopy" AND "endodontic")	33	33	13					
Scopus	"roughness" AND "endodontic"	TITLE-ABS-KEY ("roughness" AND "endodontic")	67	65	12					
Scopus	"roughness" AND sodium "hypochlorite"	TITLE-ABS-KEY ("roughness" AND "sodium" AND "hypochlorite")	1	1	1					
Scopus	"roughness" AND "ethylenediaminetetraacetic acid"	TITLE-ABS-KEY ("roughness" AND "ethylenediaminetetraacetic acid")	40	40	2					
Scopus	"sodium hypochlorite" AND "atomic force microscopy"	TITLE-ABS-KEY ("sodium hypochlorite" AND "atomic force microscopy")	80	80	9					
Scopus	"atomic force microscopy" AND "NiTi rotary instruments"	TITLE-ABS-KEY ("atomic force microscopy" AND "NiTi rotary instruments")	2	2	2					
Total records			1036	946	228	104	50	24	26	11

Table 2. K agreement calculation, Po = 0.94 (proportion of agreement), Pe = 0.6092 (agreement expected), K agreement = 0.8464 (<0 no agreement, 0.0 to 0.20 slight agreement, 0.21 to 0.40 fair agreement, 0.41 to 0.60 moderate agreement, 0.61 to 0.80 substantial agreement, and 0.81 to 1.00 almost perfect agreement). The K agreement was calculated from the 50 articles and included eleven articles with the application of the inclusion and exclusion criteria.

/	/	Reviewer 2 Include	Reviewer 2 Exclude	Reviewer 2 Unsure	Total
Reviewer 1	include	11	0	0	11
Reviewer 1	exclude	2	36	0	38
Reviewer 1	unsure	1	0	0	1
	total	14	36	0	50

3. Results

A total of 1036 records were identified on the PubMed and Scopus databases (Table 1). After screening the articles, with the restriction by year of publication (1979 to 2019), there were 946 records. With the application of the eligibility criteria (all the articles pertaining to the issue of sterilization in endodontics), there were 228 articles. There were 104 articles after eliminating overlaps. There were 50 articles that discussed the influence of sterilization procedures on the surface characteristics of endodontic instruments, and 26 that measured parameters on surface alteration.

Applying the inclusion and exclusion criteria resulted in a total of eleven articles for quantitative analysis.

Four articles were in reference to the primary outcome, eight to the secondary outcome, and five to the tertiary outcome. The entire selection and screening procedures are described in the flow chart (Figure 1).

3.1. Study Characteristics and Data Extraction

The studies included for quantitative analysis were:

- First outcome: Yılmaz et al., 2017 [9]; Spagnuolo et al., 2012 [17]; Inan et al., 2007 [10]; and Can Saglam et al., 2015 [18];
- Second outcome: Uslu et al., 2018 [19]; Can Saglam et al., 2015 [18]; Fayyad et al., 2013 [11]; Ametrano et al., 2010 [12]; Topuz et al., 2008 [20]; Cai et al., 2017 [21]; Saglam et al., 2012 [22]; and Prasad et al., 2014 [23];
- Third outcome: Uslu et al., 2018 [19]; Fayyad et al., 2013 [11]; Ametrano et al., 2010 [12]; Cai et al., 2017 [21]; and Prasad et al., 2014 [23].

The extracted data included the magazine (author, data, and journal); the endodontic instrumentation object of measurement (name, taper, and diameter at tip); the method of sterilization by heat (temperature, pressure, and time); the number autoclave cycles or irrigants; the number of instruments (control and experimental); the number of surfaces scanned by the instrument; the number of total scans; the size of the scanning surface; and the data concerning the root mean square (RMS) ± standard deviation.

The data extracted for the tree outcomes are shown in Tables 3 and 4.

3.2. Risk of Bias

The risk of bias was assessed through the Newcastle–Ottawa case-control scale. The results are reported in detail in Table 5. For each category, a value of one to three was assigned (one = low and three = high).

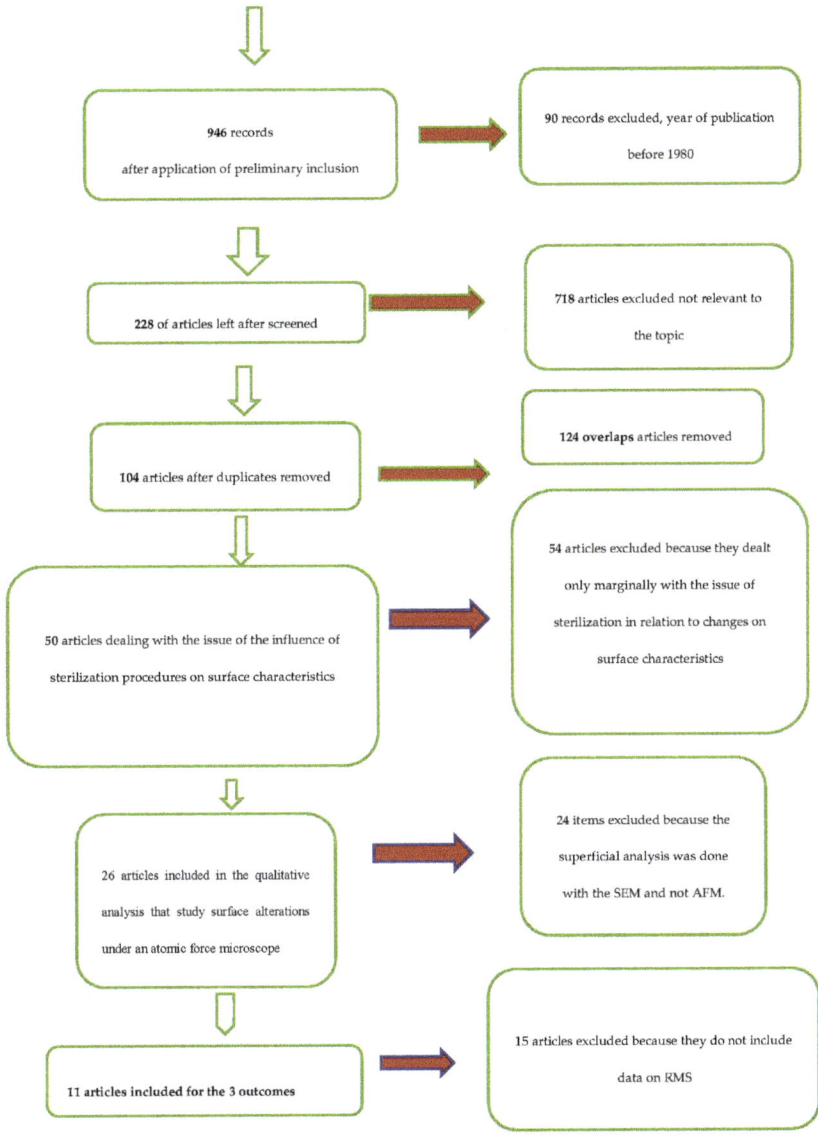

Figure 1. Flow chart of the different phases of the systematic review.

Table 3. Primary outcome (extraction of data relating to the root mean square detected on the surface of the endodontic instruments subjected to atomic force microscopy examination, with respect to control and after 5 cycles of autoclaving).

Autor, Data, Journal	Sterilization Method (Autoclave Temperature, Pressure Exposure Time)	Endodontic Instruments (Diameter and Taper at the Tip)	Autoclave Cycles	Number of Instruments	Surfaces Scanned by Instrument	Number of Total Scans	Scanning Surface	Root Mean Square (RMS) ± Standard Deviation
Yilmaz et al., 2017, Clin. Oral. Investig. [9]	Autoclave 134 °C, 30 psi for 20 min	HyFlex EDM (25/08)	0	2	15	30	5 × 5 µm	48.62 ± 7.76 nm
			5	2	15	30	5 × 5 µm	57.84 ± 6.94 nm
Spagnuolo et al., 2012, Int. Endod. J. [17]	Autoclave 121 °C, 15 psi, for 15 min	ProTaper F2 (25/08)	0	15	15	225	15 × 15 µm	203.75 ± 35.81 nm
			5	15	15	225	15 × 15 µm	715.22 nm ± 37.71
Can Saglam et al., 2015, Microsc. Res. Tech. [18]	Autoclave 121 °C for 20 min	ProTaper retreatment D1 (30/09)	0	1	11	11	2 × 2 µm	1.33 ± 0.558 nm
			5	1	11	11	2 × 2 µm	1.75 ± 0.940 nm
Inan et al., 2007, J. Endod. [10]	Autoclave 134 °C for 18 min	ProTaper F2 (25/08)	0	1	11	11	1 × 1 µm	1.46 ± 0.45 nm
			1	1	11	11	1 × 1 µm	7.29 ± 0.88 nm

Table 4. Extracted data relating to the secondary outcome and tertiary outcome, the data extracted are the root mean square (RMS), the total number of surfaces scanned, the endodontic instruments being scanned by the atomic force microscopy, and the irrigants used with the relative concentrations.

Autor, Data, Journal	Endodontic Instruments (Diameter and Taper at the Tip)	Irrigant Used (Concentration and Exposure Time)	Number of Instruments	Surfaces Scanned by Instrument	Number of Total Scans	Scanning Surface	Root Mean Square (RMS) ± Standard Deviation
Uslu et al., 2018, Microsc. Res. Tech. [19]	HyFlex EDM (25/.08)	control	4	20	80	5 × 5 μm	42.44 ± 4.51 nm
		NaOCl 5.25% for 5 min	4	20	80	5 × 5 μm	57.05 ± 8.55 nm
		EDTA 17% for 5 min	4	20	80	5 × 5 μm	60.65 ± 7.27 nm
Can Saglam et al., 2015, Microsc. Res. Tech. [18]	ProTaper retreatment D1 (30/09)	Control	1	11	11	2 × 2 μm	1.33 ± 0.558 nm
		NaOCl 2% for 5 min	1	11	11	2 × 2 μm	2.24 ± 0.555 nm
Fayyad et al., 2013, Int. Endod. J. [11]	RaCe	control	4	15	60	20 × 20 μm	83.3 ± 3.1 nm
		NaOCl 5.25% for 5 min	2	15	30	20 × 20 μm	92.3 ± 23.5 nm
		EDTA 17% for 5 min	2	15	30	20 × 20 μm	90 ± 7.5 nm
Ametrano et al., 2011, Int. Endod. J. [12]	ProTaper F2 (25/08)	control	1	20	20	1 × 1 μm	2.88 ± 0.72 nm
		NaOCl 5.25% for 5 min	1	20	20	1 × 1 μm	4.10 ± 1.13 nm
		EDTA 17% for 5 min	1	20	20	1 × 1 μm	4.79 ± 0.74 nm
Topuz et al., 2008, Oral. Surg. Oral. Med. Oral. Pathol. Oral. Radiol. Endod. [20]	RaCe rotary NiTi files (30.06)	control	1	11	11	1 × 1 μm	2.06 ± 0.49 nm
		NaOCl 5.25% for 5 min	1	11	11	1 × 1 μm	6.99 ± 2.18 nm
Saglam et al. Microsc. Res. Tech. 2012 [22]	ProTapar f3 (30.08)	control	1	12	12	5 × 5 μm	1.31 ± 0.558 nm
		NaOCl 5% for 10 min	1	12	12	5 × 5 μm	3.20 ± 1.280 nm
Prasad et al., 2014, J. Conserv. Dent. [23]	iRaCe-R3	control	1	9	9	1 × 1 μm	1.35 ± 0.29 nm
		NaOCL 5%	1	9	9	1 × 1 μm	4.74 ± 1.09 nm
		EDTA 17%	1	9	9	1 × 1 μm	3.90 ± 0.58 nm
Cai et al., 2017, Int. Endod. J. [21]	HyFlex (25.06)	control	1	15	15	1 × 1 μm	10.12 ± 1.88 nm
		NaOCl 5.25% for 10 min	1	15	15	1 × 1 μm	9.35 ± 2.05 nm
		control	1	15	15	1 × 1 μm	10.47 ± 2.34 nm
		EDTA 17% for 10 min	1	15	15	1 × 1 μm	13.88 ± 3.78 nm

Table 5. Assessment of risk of bias within the studies (Newcastle–Ottawa scale) with scores 7 to 12 = low quality, 13 to 20 = intermediate quality, and 21 to 24 = high quality.

Reference	Selection				Comparability	Exposure			Score
	Definition of Cases	Representativeness of Cases	Selection of Controls	Definition of Controls	Comparability of Cases and Controls on the Basis of the Design or Analysis	Ascertainment of Exposure	Same Method of Ascertainment for Cases and Controls	Non-Response Rate	
Cai et al., 2017 [21]	3	3	3	3	3	3	3	0	21
Prasad et al., 2014 [23]	2	2	2	2	2	2	3	0	15
Saglam et al., 2012 [22]	3	2	3	3	3	3	3	0	20
Topuz et al., 2008 [20]	3	2	3	3	3	3	3	0	20
Ametrano et al., 2011 [12]	2	2	2	2	3	3	3	0	17
Fayyad et al., 2013 [11]	2	2	2	2	2	3	3	0	16
Can Saglam et al., 2015 [18]	3	2	3	3	3	3	3	0	20
Uslu et al., 2018 [19]	3	3	3	3	3	3	3	0	21
Inan et al., 2007 [10]	3	2	3	3	3	3	3	0	20
Yılmaz et al., 2017 [9]	3	3	3	3	3	3	3	0	21
Spagnuolo et al., 2012 [17]	3	3	3	3	3	3	3	0	21

The risk of bias within the individual studies was low enough that the methods of investigation adopted for the controls were identical to the cases included in the meta-analysis. The Prasad study [23] was the only study of the exposure time of endodontic instruments to canal irrigants that was not well defined, exposing the study to a bias.

The risk of bias between the various studies was considered high, and therefore partly limited the importance of the results. The heterogeneity of the studies depended mainly on the diversity of the instruments, which were similar, in some cases, only in terms of tip diameter, taper, and type of metal alloy.

The heterogeneity of the studies was represented by funnel plots of the four outcomes, as shown in Figure 2.

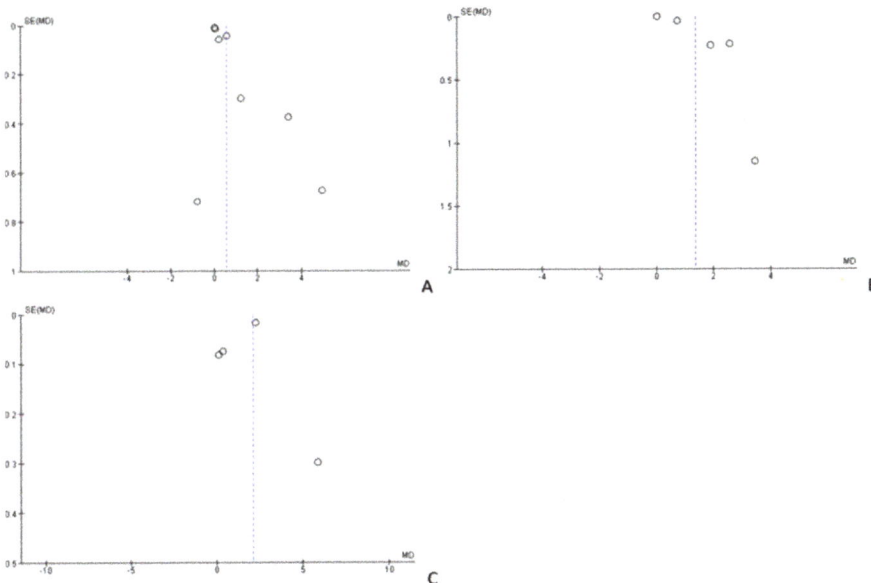

Figure 2. Funnel plots of the evaluation of heterogeneity for the (**A**) first, (**B**) second, (**C**) third outcomes.

3.3. Data Analysis

The statistical analysis of the data was performed using the Rev Manager 5.3 software (Copenhagen, 153 Denmark, The Nordic Cochrane Centre, The Nordic Cochrane Collaboration, 2014) and the results were represented by forest plots for each of the outcomes.

For the primary outcome, variations of the root mean square root (RMS) of endodontic instruments subjected to five autoclave cycles as compared with the non-autoclaved control, the comparison showed high heterogeneity of the studies, with an I2 equal to 100%. For this reason, a random effects model was used. Overall, for the primary outcome, meta-analysis was favorable for the control group. The studies that present data with a statistically significant difference are Inan et al., 2007 [10] and Spagnuolo et al., 20012 [17]. The studies by Ylmaz et al., 2018 [9] and Can Saglam et al., 2015 [22] are exactly at the center of the line of no effect. The studies by Ylzam and Can Saglam are exactly at the center of the line of no effect, however, the remaining two studies are favorable for the group subjected to control, their confidence intervals do not intercept the line of no effect (Figure 3).

autoclave
Control
Mean Difference
Mean Difference
Study or Subgroup Mean SD Total Mean SD Total Weight IV, Random, 95% CI
IV, Random, 95% CI
Can Saglam 2015 0.4375 0.235 11 0.3325 0.1395 11 25.2% 0.10 [-0.06, 0.27]
Inan I 2007 7.29 0.88 11 1.46 0.45 11 24.3% 5.83 [5.25, 6.41]
Spagnuolo 2012 3.17875 0.1676 225 0.9055 0.19515 225 25.3% 2.27 [2.24, 2.31]
Yilmaz 2018 2.3136 0.2776 30 1.9448 0.3104 30 25.2% 0.37 [0.22, 0.52]
Total (95% CI) 277 277 100.0% 2.11 [0.65, 3.57]
Heterogeneity: Tau² = 2.19; Chi² = 1363.03, df = 3 (P < 0.00001); I² = 100%
Test for overall effect: Z = 2.83 (P = 0.005)
-10 -5 0 5 10
[autoclave] [control]

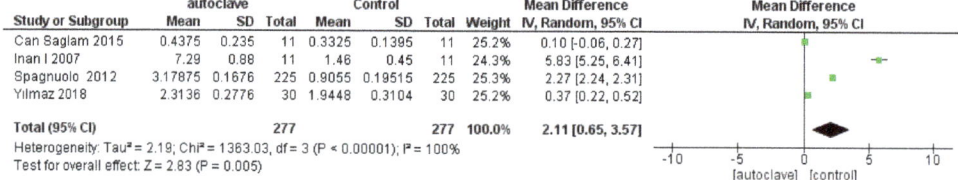

Figure 3. Forest plot of the random effects model of the meta-analysis of the primary outcome.

For the secondary outcome, variations of the root mean square (RMS) of endodontic instruments exposed to sodium hypochlorite 5% as compared with the control group, the comparison showed high heterogeneity among the studies, with an I2 equal to 98%. For this reason, for the second outcome, a random effects model was applied to avoid minimizing the roles of smaller-dimension studies. For the second outcome, the forest plot is in favor of the subject group control.

The studies that reported statistically significant data in favor of the control group are Ametrano, 2011; Prasad, 2014; Topuz, 2008; and Uslu, 2018. The Cai's study was the only study that was in favor of the group subjected to sodium hypochlorite, even though its confidence interval crosses the line of no effect. The other studies report statistically insignificant data (Figure 4).

NaOCl
Control
Mean Difference
Mean Difference
Study or Subgroup Mean SD Total Mean SD Total Weight IV, Random, 95% CI
IV, Random, 95% CI
Ametrano 2011 4.1 1.13 20 2.88 0.72 20 7.4% 1.22 [0.63, 1.81]
Cai 2017 9.35 2.05 15 10.12 1.88 15 1.8% -0.77 [-2.18, 0.64]
Can Saglam 2015 0.56 0.13875 11 0.3325 0.1395 11 20.0% 0.23 [0.11, 0.34]
Fayyad 2013 0.23075 0.05875 30 0.20825 0.00775 60 21.5% 0.02 [0.00, 0.04]
Prasad 2014 4.74 1.09 9 1.35 0.29 9 5.3% 3.39 [2.65, 4.13]
Saglam 2012 0.128 0.0512 12 0.0524 0.02232 12 21.4% 0.08 [0.04, 0.11]
Topuz 2008 6.99 2.18 11 2.06 0.49 11 2.0% 4.93 [3.61, 6.25]
Uslu 2018 2.282 0.342 80 1.6976 0.1804 80 20.7% 0.58 [0.50, 0.67]
Total (95% CI) 188 218 100.0% 0.54 [0.35, 0.74]
Heterogeneity: Tau² = 0.05; Chi² = 314.28, df = 7 (P < 0.00001); I² = 98%
Test for overall effect: Z = 5.42 (P < 0.00001)
-4 -2 0 2 4
Favours [NaOCL] Favours [control]

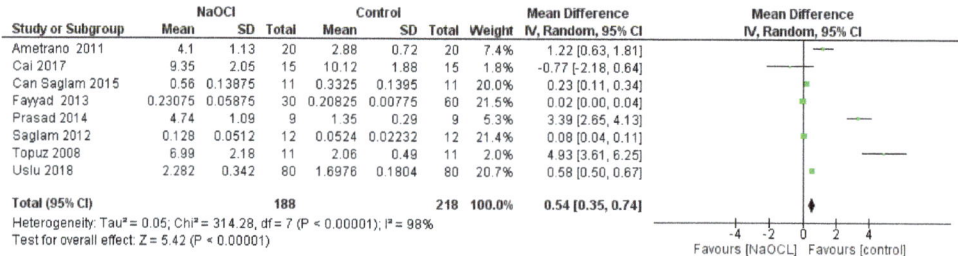

Figure 4. Forest plot of the random effects model of the meta-analysis of the secondary outcome.

For the tertiary outcome, variations of the root mean square (RMS) of the endodontic instruments exposed to EDTA 10% as compared with the control group, the comparison showed high heterogeneity between the studies, with an I2 of 99%, and therefore a random effects model was applied. For the tertiary outcome, the forest plot is in favor of the control group except for the study by Fayyad which is positioned in the line of no effect (Figure 5).

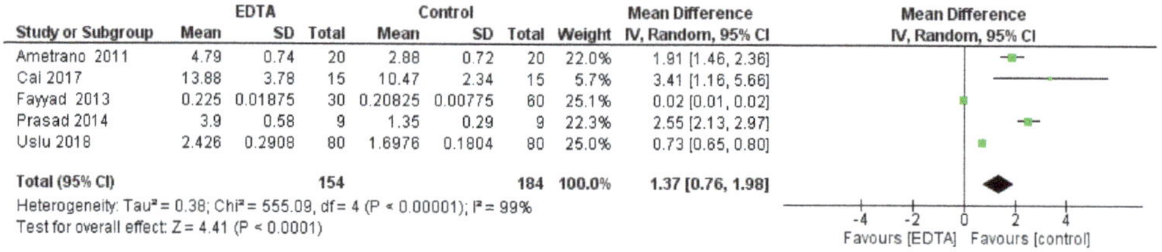

EDTA
Control
Mean Difference
Mean Difference
Study or Subgroup Mean SD Total Mean SD Total Weight IV, Random, 95% CI
IV, Random, 95% CI
Ametrano 2011 4.79 0.74 20 2.88 0.72 20 22.0% 1.91 [1.46, 2.36]
Cai 2017 13.88 3.78 15 10.47 2.34 15 5.7% 3.41 [1.16, 5.66]
Fayyad 2013 0.225 0.01875 30 0.20825 0.00775 60 25.1% 0.02 [0.01, 0.02]
Prasad 2014 3.9 0.58 9 1.35 0.29 9 22.3% 2.55 [2.13, 2.97]
Uslu 2018 2.426 0.2908 80 1.6976 0.1804 80 25.0% 0.73 [0.65, 0.80]
Total (95% CI) 154 184 100.0% 1.37 [0.76, 1.98]
Heterogeneity: Tau² = 0.38; Chi² = 555.09, df = 4 (P < 0.00001); I² = 99%
Test for overall effect: Z = 4.41 (P < 0.0001)
-4 -2 0 2 4
Favours [EDTA] Favours [control]

Figure 5. Forest plot of the random effects model of the meta-analysis of the tertiary outcome.

4. Discussion

The results of the meta-analysis for the three outcomes are in agreement in establishing that the superficial alterations induced by autoclave, from the sodium hypochlorite and from the EDTA, are statistically significant surface alterations that represent points where instrument fractures can be triggered. In addition, the alterations induced on the surface analyzed by SEM and AFM show that the alterations can also be expressed on the cutting surface, altering, in a pejorative sense, the cutting efficacy.

For the first outcome, the studies, in the literature, that supported a statistically significant alteration are:

1. In 2007, Inan reported statistically significant data for all the instruments of the ProTaper series (S1, S2, F1, F2), and reported that the superficial deterioration induced by the autoclave is greater for ProTaper finished than for ProTaper shaping;
2. In 2012, Spagnuolo confirmed, in agreement with Inan's data, that multiple cycles (autoclave sterilization) modified the surface topography and chemical composition of conventional NiTi (F2 ProTaper) and TiN-coated (alpha kit) instruments, in a statistically significant way (after five autoclave cycles).

Sodium hypochlorite certainly alters the surface of NiTi instruments and innumerable studies are in agreement such as Uslu et al., 2018 [19]; Ametrano et al., 2010 [12]; Topuz et al., 2008 [20]; and Prasad et al., 2014 [23]. Furthermore, a study conducted by Yokoyama et al., 2004 [24] stated that the action of sodium hypochlorite causes a worsening of the surface in endodontic instruments that facilitates their rupture following flexor and torsional stress.

The statistical analysis, in a similar way but with fewer studies, also confirms that the EDTA determines an increase in surface irregularities in a statistically significant way, and studies that confirm it after 10 min of exposure are well highlighted in the forest plot (Figure 5). Studies that are in contrast to the present meta-analysis report conflicting data regarding the action of EDTA on the surface. It seems that for exposures less than 5 min they do not alter the surface, however, according to Bonaccorsa et al. [25], a passivation phenomenon could lead to the creation of a complex between the metallic ions and the EDTA at a PH lower than four which renders the instrument resistant.

5. Conclusions

In conclusion, based on the present systematic analysis we affirm that autoclave induces a statistically significant corrosive phenomena, called micropitting, after five cycles of autoclave and determined by the heat, and comparatively, hypochlorite determines corrosion after only 5 min of exposure and EDTA after 10 min of exposure.

Superficial alterations, which are widely discussed in the literature, can determine the triggering of fractures in instruments subjected to cyclic fatigue and torsional fatigue. Therefore, it is important for endodontist to have knowledge of such corrosive phenomena, induced by irrigants such as sodium hypochlorite and EDTA, on instruments that can be reused and autoclaved.

Author Contributions: Conceptualization, M.D., D.S., and B.R.; methodology, K.Z. and M.D.; software, M.A. validation, M.D., and L.L.M.; formal analysis, D.S., M.D., and V.C.; investigation, L.L. and M.D.; resources, L.L.M.; data curation, E.L. and M.D.; writing—original draft preparation, M.D.; writing—review and editing, M.D., L.L.M., L.L.R., D.C., and F.M.

Funding: This research received no external funding.

Acknowledgments: All the acknowledgements go to Lorenzo Lo Muzio, Director of the Dental Clinic and President of the Department of Clinical and Experimental Medicine of the University of Foggia, who gave fundamental technical support in the writing of this article.

Conflicts of Interest: The authors declare no conflict of interest.

References

1. Inan, U.; Keskin, C. Torsional Resistance of ProGlider, Hyflex EDM, and One G Glide Path Instruments. *J. Endod.* **2019**. [CrossRef]
2. Troiano, G.; Dioguardi, M.; Cocco, A.; Zhurakivska, K.; Ciavarella, D.; Muzio, L.L. Increase in [corrected] the glyde path diameter improves the centering ability of F6 Skytaper. *Eur. J. Dent.* **2018**, *12*, 89–93. [CrossRef] [PubMed]
3. Laneve, E.; Raddato, B.; Dioguardi, M.; Di Gioia, G.; Troiano, G.; Lo Muzio, L. Sterilisation in Dentistry: A Review of the Literature. *Int. J. Dent.* **2019**, *2019*, 6507286. [CrossRef] [PubMed]
4. Dioguardi, M.; Di Gioia, G.; Illuzzi, G.; Laneve, E.; Cocco, A.; Troiano, G. Endodontic irrigants: Different methods to improve efficacy and related problems. *Eur. J. Dent.* **2018**, *12*, 459–466. [CrossRef] [PubMed]
5. Berutti, E.; Angelini, E.; Rigolone, M.; Migliaretti, G.; Pasqualini, D. Influence of sodium hypochlorite on fracture properties and corrosion of ProTaper Rotary instruments. *Int. Endod. J.* **2006**, *39*, 693–699. [CrossRef] [PubMed]
6. Dioguardi, M.; Sovereto, D.; Aiuto, R.; Laino, L.; Illuzzi, G.; Laneve, E.; Raddato, B.; Caponio, V.C.A.; Dioguardi, A.; Zhurakivska, K.; et al. Effects of Hot Sterilization on Torsional Properties of Endodontic Instruments: Systematic Review with Meta-Analysis. *Materials* **2019**, *12*, 2190. [CrossRef] [PubMed]
7. Shen, Y.; Coil, J.M.; McLean, A.G.; Hemerling, D.L.; Haapasalo, M. Defects in nickel-titanium instruments after clinical use. Part 5: Single use from endodontic specialty practices. *J. Endod.* **2009**, *35*, 1363–1367. [CrossRef]
8. Ozyurek, T.; Yilmaz, K.; Uslu, G.; Plotino, G. The effect of root canal preparation on the surface roughness of WaveOne and WaveOne Gold files: Atomic force microscopy study. *Restor. Dent. Endod.* **2018**, *43*, e10. [CrossRef]
9. Yilmaz, K.; Uslu, G.; Ozyurek, T. Effect of multiple autoclave cycles on the surface roughness of HyFlex CM and HyFlex EDM files: An atomic force microscopy study. *Clin. Oral Investig.* **2018**, *22*, 2975–2980. [CrossRef]
10. Inan, U.; Aydin, C.; Uzun, O.; Topuz, O.; Alacam, T. Evaluation of the surface characteristics of used and new ProTaper Instruments: An atomic force microscopy study. *J. Endod.* **2007**, *33*, 1334–1337. [CrossRef]
11. Fayyad, D.M.; Mahran, A.H. Atomic force microscopic evaluation of nanostructure alterations of rotary NiTi instruments after immersion in irrigating solutions. *Int. Endod. J.* **2014**, *47*, 567–573. [CrossRef] [PubMed]
12. Ametrano, G.; D'Anto, V.; Di Caprio, M.P.; Simeone, M.; Rengo, S.; Spagnuolo, G. Effects of sodium hypochlorite and ethylenediaminetetraacetic acid on rotary nickel-titanium instruments evaluated using atomic force microscopy. *Int. Endod. J.* **2011**, *44*, 203–209. [CrossRef] [PubMed]
13. Casella, G.; Rosalbino, F. Corrosion behaviour of NiTi endodontic instrument. *Corros. Eng. Sci. Technol.* **2011**, *46*, 521–523. [CrossRef]
14. Razavian, H.; Iranmanesh, P.; Mojtahedi, H.; Nazeri, R. Effect of Autoclave Cycles on Surface Characteristics of S-File Evaluated by Scanning Electron Microscopy. *Iran. Endod. J.* **2016**, *11*, 29–32. [CrossRef]
15. Higgins, J.P.T.; Green, S. *Cochrane Collaboration. Cochrane Handbook for Systematic Reviews of Interventions*; Wiley-Blackwell: Chichester, UK; Hoboken, NJ, USA, 2008; 649p.
16. Lo, C.K.; Mertz, D.; Loeb, M. Newcastle-Ottawa Scale: Comparing reviewers' to authors' assessments. *BMC Med. Res. Methodol.* **2014**, *14*, 45. [CrossRef] [PubMed]
17. Spagnuolo, G.; Ametrano, G.; D'Anto, V.; Rengo, C.; Simeone, M.; Riccitiello, F.; Amato, M. Effect of autoclaving on the surfaces of TiN -coated and conventional nickel-titanium rotary instruments. *Int. Endod. J.* **2012**, *45*, 1148–1155. [CrossRef] [PubMed]
18. Can Saglam, B.; Gorgul, G. Evaluation of surface alterations in different retreatment nickel-titanium files: AFM and SEM study. *Microsc. Res. Tech.* **2015**, *78*, 356–362. [CrossRef]
19. Uslu, G.; Ozyurek, T.; Yilmaz, K. Effect of Sodium Hypochlorite and EDTA on Surface Roughness of HyFlex CM and HyFlex EDM Files. *Microsc. Res. Tech.* **2018**, *81*, 1406–1411. [CrossRef]
20. Topuz, O.; Aydin, C.; Uzun, O.; Inan, U.; Alacam, T.; Tunca, Y.M. Structural effects of sodium hypochlorite solution on RaCe rotary nickel-titanium instruments: An atomic force microscopy study. *Oral Surg. Oral Med. Oral Pathol. Oral Radiol. Endod.* **2008**, *105*, 661–665. [CrossRef]
21. Cai, J.J.; Tang, X.N.; Ge, J.Y. Effect of irrigation on surface roughness and fatigue resistance of controlled memory wire nickel-titanium instruments. *Int. Endod. J.* **2017**, *50*, 718–724. [CrossRef]

22. Saglam, B.C.; Kocak, S.; Kocak, M.M.; Topuz, O. Effects of irrigation solutions on the surface of ProTaper instruments: A microscopy study. *Microsc. Res. Tech.* **2012**, *75*, 1534–1538. [CrossRef] [PubMed]
23. Prasad, P.S.; Sam, J.E.; Arvind Kumar, K. The effect of 5% sodium hypochlorite, 17% EDTA and triphala on two different rotary Ni-Ti instruments: An AFM and EDS analysis. *J. Conserv. Dent.* **2014**, *17*, 462–466. [CrossRef] [PubMed]
24. Yokoyama, K.; Kancko, K.; Yabuta, E.; Asaoka, K.; Sakai, J. Fracture of nickel-titanium superelastic alloy in sodium hypochlorite solution. *Mater. Sci. Eng. A* **2004**, *369*, 43–48. [CrossRef]
25. Bonaccorso, A.; Tripi, T.R.; Rondelli, G.; Condorelli, G.G.; Cantatore, G.; Schafer, E. Pitting corrosion resistance of nickel-titanium rotary instruments with different surface treatments in seventeen percent ethylenediaminetetraacetic Acid and sodium chloride solutions. *J. Endod.* **2008**, *34*, 208–211. [CrossRef]

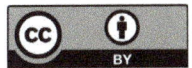

© 2019 by the authors. Licensee MDPI, Basel, Switzerland. This article is an open access article distributed under the terms and conditions of the Creative Commons Attribution (CC BY) license (http://creativecommons.org/licenses/by/4.0/).

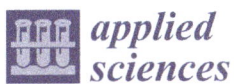

Article

Influence of Myeloperoxidase Levels on Periodontal Disease: An Applied Clinical Study

Alessandro Polizzi *, Salvatore Torrisi, Simona Santonocito, Mattia Di Stefano, Francesco Indelicato and Antonino Lo Giudice

Department of General Surgery and Surgical-Medical Specialties, School of Dentistry, University of Catania, AOU Policlinico—P.O. Vittorio Emanuele, Via Plebiscito 628, 95124 Catania, Italy; ture_torrisi@hotmail.it (S.T.); simonasantonocito.93@gmail.com (S.S.); mattiadistefano@live.it (M.D.S.); indelicato@policlinico.unict.it (F.I.); nino.logiudice@gmail.com (A.L.G.)
* Correspondence: alexpoli345@gmail.com; Tel./Fax: +39-0957435359

Received: 26 January 2020; Accepted: 3 February 2020; Published: 4 February 2020

Abstract: In this trial, we evaluated the influence on plasma and salivary myeloperoxidase (MPO) levels of periodontal health, coronary heart disease (CHD), periodontitis, or both periodontitis and CHD. Clinical and periodontal parameters were collected from periodontitis patients (n = 31), CHD patients (n = 31), patients with both periodontitis and CHD (n = 31), and from healthy patients (n = 31) together with saliva and plasma samples. The median concentrations of salivary and plasma MPO were statistically higher in the CHD patients [plasma: 26.2 (18.2–34.4) ng/mg; saliva 83.2 (77.4–101.5) ng/mL, $p < 0.01$] and in the periodontitis plus CHD patients [plasma: 27.8 (22.5–35.7) ng/mg; saliva 85.6 (76.5–106.7) ng/mL, $p < 0.001$] with respect to periodontitis and control patients. Through a univariate regression analysis, c-reactive protein (CRP) and CHD (both $p < 0.001$) and periodontitis ($p = 0.024$) were statistically correlated with MPO in plasma. The multivariate regression analysis demonstrated that only CRP was statistically the predictor of MPO in plasma ($p < 0.001$). The multivariate regression analysis in saliva demonstrated that, regarding MPO levels the only predictors were CRP ($p < 0.001$) and total cholesterol ($p = 0.035$). The present study evidenced that subjects with CHD and periodontitis plus CHD had higher plasma and salivary levels of MPO compared to subjects with periodontitis and healthy controls.

Keywords: myeloperoxidase; periodontitis; cardiovascular disease; applied model

1. Introduction

Periodontal disease is a common oral inflammatory multifactorial disease that causes the disruption of the periodontium and the tissues that support the tooth, such as bone and cementum main caused by oral bacteria, that ultimately leads to the loss of the tooth [1]. Almost all adults in the USA present periodontal disease forms and nearly ten percent of the population worldwide express severe type of periodontal disease [2,3].

More recently, observational reports have shown a correlation between periodontal disease and cardiovascular disease, such as stroke, heart disease and endothelial dysfunction [4,5]. Moreover, some studies demonstrated a specific correlation among periodontal disease and an augmented risk of stroke [6] and, coronary heart disease (CHD) [7,8].

The pathogenesis of periodontal disease includes inflammatory and bacteria responses which may determine an increased host response subsequent to the presence of pathogenic oral biofilm in gingival tissues [9]. More specifically, periodontal disease has been correlated with an increase of levels of some systemic inflammatory mediators in serum, such as prostaglandin, interleukin 1 (IL-1), IL-6, and C-reactive protein (CRP) [10].

Myeloperoxidase (MPO) is one of the more mediators expressed within tissues during the progression of inflammation [11]. It was demonstrated that MPO, secreted by endothelial cells after exposure to pathogenic bacteria, represents a potent mediator of vascular inflammation and a vasoconstrictor [12].

In this regard, it has been shown that several proinflammatory cytokines, including IL-1, -6, and -8, have been reported to upregulate the secretion of MPO [13]. The expression of MPO was strongly associated in the gingival tissue and endothelial cells during periodontitis [14]. More specifically, a clinical study found that, in gingival crevicular fluid, MPO increased with the progression of the periodontitis, and also that MPO was involved in the regulation of IL-1b expression in gingival tissues [15,16].

During the last few decades, several studies have analyzed the association between periodontal disease endothelial dysfunction, and increased risk of CHD and cardiovascular disease (CVD) [17,18]. More specifically, it has been supposed that the inflammatory mediators that are present and released during the active phase of periodontal disease such as CRP, interleukins, prostaglandins, and metalloproteases, can negatively influence the release of nitric oxide (NO) [19]. The altered release of NO can affect the endothelium which in turn regulates vascular tone, and, finally, dysfunction of the endothelium and enhanced risk of CVD [20,21]. For these causes, there is growing interest to investigate some other oral mediators that can regulate and impact the subclinical endothelial dysfunctions as an early sign of augmented risk of CHD and CVD. In this regard, a correlation between high proportion of MPO, CRP, and endothelial dysfunction was recently reported [22,23].

The production of NO at local level has been shown to be fundamental in the aetiology and progression of periodontitis. The increment and reduction of NO metabolites in saliva production in periodontal tissue against periodontopathogenic microbiota during periodontitis have been demonstrated to be correlated endothelial dysfunction [24,25]. Furthermore, it has been reported that MPO plays an important role in the reduction of NO synthase especially during periodontitis [26].

Based on these findings, the aims of this trial were to consider a possible association of periodontitis, CVD, or both periodontitis plus CVD on serum and salivary MPO. Futhermore, we analyzed the possible correlation between MPO in serum and saliva and if serum CRP mediated the association between salivary or serum MPO levels.

2. Materials and Methods

2.1. Study Design

For the present study, 311 healthy controls and patients with periodontitis or CHD were chosen at the School of Odontostomatology of the University of Catania, Italy, from October 2018 to December 2019. Patients were chosen in a specific range of age (35–65 years old) and on gender in order to have similar proportion of patients in each category characterized by the selection variable. 50% of the patients and controls were males with 45–54 year of age.

The study was performed following the 2016 revision of the Helsinki declaration on medical research. Ethical approval was obtained by the local International Review Board (IRB) (#18-18). The study was registered at clinicaltrials.gov (NCT04152023). An informed written consent was obtained from each enrolled patient. The trial was performed in accordance to the guidelines for the strengthening of reporting of observational studies (STROBE) [27].

The inclusion criteria for the subjects enrolled in the periodontitis group were: (1) at least 16 teeth, (2) at least of 40% of periodontal sites with clinical attachment level (CAL) ≥ 2 mm and probing depth (PD) ≥ 4 mm [28]; (3) at least one periodontal site with ≥ 2 mm of crestal alveolar bone loss confirmed on digital periapical x-rays; (4) at least ≥ 40% sites with bleeding on probing (BOP) [29]. Healthy controls had any systemic disorder, at least ≤ 10% sites with BOP, and no periodontal sites with PD or CAL ≥ 4 mm, or x-ray signs of bone loss.

For the CVD group, the inclusion criteria were: at least ≥18 years; a diagnosis of CVD with ≥50% of stenosis of at least one coronary artery verified by coronary angiography, or past or current percutaneous coronary intervention [30]. Each type of previous disease, taking drugs, or previous CVD exams (e.g., electrocardiography, etc.) were recorded. In all patients, the diagnosis of CVD was performed by the same operator from medical record information. For the periodontitis plus CVD subjects the inclusion criteria were the same of the single disease (periodontitis and CVD).

The exclusion criteria of all subjects, were (1) consumption of contraceptive drugs; (2) consumption of antibiotics, anti-inflammatory or immunosuppressive drugs during the three months previous the trial; (3) presence of gestation or suction; (4) intake of alcohol; (5) anesthetic allergy; (6) intake of nifedipine, hydantoin or cyclosporin a drugs; (7) any type of periodontal treatment in the three months before baseline.

Then, 187 subjects were left out from the study because they did not meet the inclusion criteria (n = 129), failed to join in the study (n = 37), or were lost at the first assessment (n = 21). For these reasons, for the present study, 31 healthy subjects, 31 periodontitis patients, 31 CHD patients, and 31 patients with both diseases (periodontitis plus CHD) were enrolled in the end (Figure 1).

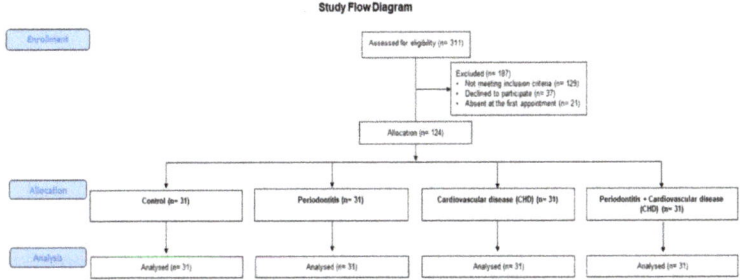

Figure 1. Flowchart of the study.

In each patient, every demographic characteristic (such as educational level) and demographic indices such as age, gender, body mass index (BMI), diabetes and other systemic events were recorded together with the type of drug taken. Diabetes was recorded on the patient's medical story or on fasting blood glucose ≥125 mg/dL. The BMI was recorded by calculating the patient's weight divided by the square of his height in kg/m^2. All enrolled subjects were also classified on their smoking history, such as normal smokers, ex-smokers (subjects who have not smoked for ≥5 years), and non-smokers.

The periodontal evaluation comprised clinical attachment loss (CAL), probing depth (PD), bleeding on probing (BOP), and plaque score (PI) [31]. CAL was verified, such as PD plus gingival recession using the cementoenamel junction as a reference. All periodontal indexes were registered, in all patients, by two independent calibrated examiners (a principal examiner and a control examiner), exonerated in the subsequent study steps, using a periodontal probe (UNC-15, Hu-Friedy, Chicago, IL, USA).

It was assessed the inter- and intra-examiner reliability for PD and CAL through the Intraclass Correlation Coefficient (ICC) analysis. The obtained inter-examiner reliability was in agreement for PD (ICC= 0.819) and CAL (ICC = 0.832) with a good degree of reliability. The intra-examiner reliability of PD and CAL was done only on 24 subjects (six random subjects per group) for both examiners. For the first examiner, the intra-examiner reliability presented an agreement for PD (ICC = 0.819) and CAL (ICC = 0.808); for the second examiner, the intra-examiner reliability was good for both PD (ICC = 0.818) and CAL (ICC = 0.801). All periodontal indexes were registered, in each enrolled subject, at six sites in each tooth.

A power analysis was executed in order to evaluate the sample size needed for the study. The sample size was determined considering four groups: an effect size of 0.29 for MPO (primary outcome chosen), a two-sided significance level of 0.05, a standard deviation of 1.5 [23], and a power level of 80%. It was established that would be required around 28 patients per group, with a total number of 114 patients required to obtain a power level of 80%. a total of 124 patients were enrolled, so the study power was 81%. Power and sample size calculation was performed with statistical software (G*Power version 3.1.9.4, Universitat Dusseldorf, Germany).

2.2. Evaluation of Salivary and Serum MPO

All serum and saliva samples were collected on an in all patients between 8:00 and 10:00 a.m., before the periodontal examination, on the same day by the same examiner. All enrolled subjects were requested to refrain from drinking, eating, chewing, brushing their teeth, or other oral hygiene maneuvers in the 12 h preceding the sampling of serum and saliva.

For the collection of serum, a venous blood sample was taken which, after the collection, was immediately cooled with ice and centrifuged at 4 °C (800× g for 10 min). For the collection of saliva samples, the enrolled patients were asked to moisten by chewing a cotton roll for two minutes using the salivette method (Sarsted, Verona, Italy). Subsequently, the saliva sample in each patient was instantaneously centrifuged at 4 °C (1000× g for 2 min). Both saliva and serum samples were stored at −20 °C.

Magnetic bead-based luminex assay (R&D Systems, Minneapolis, MN, and Sigma-Aldrich, Saint Louis, MO, USA) were used to detect serum and salivary concentrations of MPO, following the manufacturers' instructions. Levels of hs-CRP were calculated using a nephelometric assay kit. Levels of hs-CRP >3 mg/L were related to an augmented CVD risk. Routine methods were applied to assess glucose and plasma lipids levels.

2.3. Statistical Analysis

Median, 25%, and 75% percentile were used to express numerical variables while number and % were used to express categorical variables. Nearly all of the variables analyzed (e.g., fasting glucose, triglycerides, all periodontal index) did not have normal distribution, as confirmed by Kolmogorov–Smirnov test. Only age, BMI, and salivary and serum MPO were normally distributed; for this reason, nonparametric tests were used to analyze all data in the present analysis [32]. More specifically, to confront all numerical variables in the 4 groups of patients, was applied the Kruskal Wallis test while the Mann Whitney test was applied to obtain the two-by-two comparisons. Bonferroni's correction was applied for numerous evaluations; the α level of 0.050 was split by the potential comparisons (n = 6), and the adjusted significance level equalled 0.008 (0.050/6).

The *p*-trend analysis for salivary and serum and MPO levels was obtained using the Jonckheere–Terpstra Test to evaluate whether MPO levels were statistically augmented in the four analyzed groups. To asses any significant interdependence between MPO in saliva and serum and hs-CRP, the Spearman correlation test was used.

Moreover, a univariate and multivariable linear regression analysis were applied in all enrolled patients to evaluate the dependence of MPO levels in serum and saliva (which resulted normally distributed) on possibly explicative outcomes such as sex, education, age, socioeconomic status (SES), triglycerides, total cholesterol, BMI, CRP, and CVD drugs (yes/no). In the multivariate final model, sex, age, and education SES were incorporated such as possible confounders, and tested to analyze if CHD, periodontitis, and hs-CRP influenced MPO in serum. For the evaluation of MPO in saliva, the same analysis was performed using salivary MPO levels as an outcome. All statistical analyses were executed using statistical software (SPSS 22.0 for Windows package, SPS srl, Bologna, Italy). a *p*-value < 0.05 was set such as significant.

3. Results

The demographic and serological characteristics of the enrolled patients are shown in Table 1. All groups were matched for age and sex, and they did not presented any statistically significant differences regarding education levels, smoking, BMI, and serological features (Table 1).

Table 1. Sample characteristics of enrolled patients. Data are represented as median (25th; 75th percentiles) or number with percentage. * $p < 0.001$ and ** $p < 0.001$ significant differences vs. healthy subjects computed by the Mann Whitney test. §§ $p < 0.001$ significant differences vs. periodontitis patients calculated by the Mann Whitney test. # $p < 0.008$ significant differences vs. coronary heart disease (CHD) patients calculated by the Mann Whitney test.

	Controls (N = 31)	Periodontitis (N = 31)	CVD (N = 31)	Periodontitis + CVD (N = 31)
Age (years)	52 (48; 56)	53 (47; 57)	52 (46; 58)	53 (47; 56)
Gender (male/female)	15/16	16/15	14/17	16/15
Education level				
Primary school, n (%)	11 (35.4)	12 (38.7)	11 (35.4)	12 (38.7)
High school, n (%)	14 (45.1)	13 (41.9)	15 (48.3)	14 (45.1)
College/university, n (%)	6 (19.3)	6 (19.3)	5 (16.1)	5 (16.1)
Body mass index (kg/m^2)	24.4 (21.8; 27.8)	23.9 (22.4; 26.4)	24.8 (21.6; 27.1)	24.5 (22.3; 26.1)
Fasting glucose (mg/dl)	87.9 (82.1; 93.2)	88.7 (82.3; 105.3)	88.1 (80.6; 114.6)	91.1 (85.1; 109.2)
Smokers, n (%)	2 (6.4)	3 (9.6)	2 (6.4)	2 (9.6)
Never smokers, n (%)	27 (88.2)	27 (85.2)	28 (88.2)	26 (85.2)
Past smokers, n (%)	2 (6.4)	1 (3.2)	1 (3.2)	3 (9.6)
Current smokers, n (%)	2 (6.4)	3 (6.4)	2 (6.4)	2 (6.4)
Comorbidities				
Diabetes, n (%)	-	3 (9.6) **	2 (6.4) **	2 (9.6) **
Previous CVD				
Atrial fibrillation, n (%)	-	-	6 (19.3) **,§§	5 (16.1) **,§§
Angina pectoris, n (%)	-	-	12 (38.7) **,§§	13 (41.9) **,§§
Stroke, n (%)	-	-	5 (16.1) **,§§	7 (22.6) **,§§
Heart failure, n (%)	-	-	6 (19.3) **,§§	5 (16.1) **,§§
Antihypertensive, n (%)	-	-	10 (32.2) **,§§	10 (32.2) **,§§
Statins, n (%)	-	-	10 (32.2) **,§§	9 (29) **,§§
Low-dose aspirin, n (%)	-	-	7 (22.6) **,§§	7 (22.6) **,§§
Beta blockers, n (%)	-	-	6 (19.3) **,§§	8 (25.8) **,§§
hs-CRP (mg/L)	2.5 (2.1; 2.9)	3.1 (2.5; 3.9) *	5.6 (4.8; 6.2) **	6.7 (5.8; 7.1) **,§§,#
Total cholesterol (mg/dl)	162 (139; 181)	164 (133; 181)	173 (139; 197)	176 (178; 201)
Triglycerids (mg/dl)	121 (91; 145)	102 (66; 128)	141 (122; 166)	139 (103; 158)

Compared to healthy controls, patients with periodontitis, CDH and a combination of periodontitis and CVD presented a higher value of hs-CRP ($p < 0.001$). Moreover, patients with CHD and periodontitis plus CHD presented no significant differences regarding past CVD events.

In Table 2 are represented dental characteristics of all enrolled patients. Compared with CHD and control patients, subjects with periodontitis and periodontitis plus CVD showed higher periodontal parameters (CAL, PD, BOP, PI) and smaller number of teeth ($p < 0.001$) (Table 2).

Table 2. Periodontal characteristics of enrolled patients. Data are represented as median (25th; 75th percentile). CAL, clinical attachment level; PD, probing pocket depth; BOP, bleeding on probing; PI, plaque index. ** $p < 0.001$ significant differences vs. control subjects. §§ $p < 0.001$ significant differences vs. periodontitis patients. ## $p < 0.001$ significant differences vs. CHD patients.

	Controls (N = 31)	Periodontitis (N = 31)	CVD (N = 31)	Periodontitis + CVD (N = 31)
N° of teeth	26 (21; 27)	20 (15; 21)**	23 (19; 26) **,§§	18 (12; 20) **,##
CAL (mm)	1 (0.9; 1.3)	3.6 (3.1; 4.2) **	2 (1.8; 2.4) **,§§	3.4 (3; 4.1) **,##
CAL 4–5 mm (% sites)	-	38.7 (35.4; 42.9) **	-	40.6 (35.5; 46.1) **,##
CAL ≥6 mm (% sites)	-	18.7 (19.6; 22.3) **	-	17.4 (15.8; 22.7) **,##
PD (mm)	1.5 (1.3; 1.9)	4.4 (3.7; 4.6) **	2.1 (1.8; 2.4) **,§§	3.9 (3.7; 4.4) **,##
PD 4–5 mm (% sites)	-	40.9 (38.6; 45.7) **	-	44.1 (42.7; 55.3) **,##
PD ≥6 mm (% sites)	-	23.1 (19.8; 25.2) **	-	22.7 (20.3; 26.5) **,§§,##
BOP (%)	7.9 (6.5; 8.3)	41.2 (34.3; 46.5) **	8.1 (6.4; 8.9) **,§§	42.3 (41.5; 50.1) **,§§,##
Rx alveolar bone loss (mm)	0.2 (0.1; 0.5)	2.9 (2.5; 3.4) **	0.3 (0.2; 0.9) **,§§	3.3 (2.1; 4.6) **,##
PI (%)	6.5 (4.7; 9.3)	35.4 (31.7; 37.9) **	11.7 (9.1; 12.8) **,§§	32.4 (27.2; 36.1) **,##

Figure 2 represents median (25th; 75th percentile) values of MPO levels in saliva and serum of all enrolled patients. Compared to control subjects, patients with CVD ($p < 0.01$) and with periodontitis plus CVD ($p < 0.001$) had higher median concentrations of MPO in saliva and serum. More specifically, in comparison with periodontitis subjects, patients with periodontitis plus CVD presented increased salivary and serum concentrations of MPO ($p < 0.01$) (Figure 2).

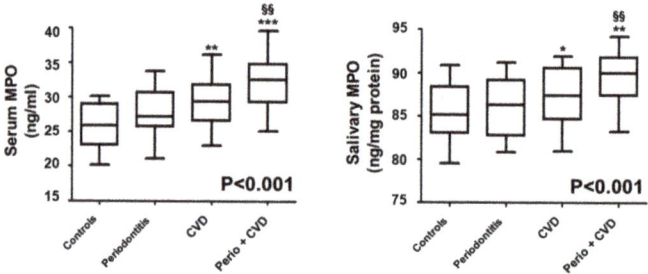

Figure 2. Median values (25%; 75% percentiles) of coronary heart disease (MPO) in saliva and serum. * $p < 0.05$, ** $p < 0.01$ and *** $p < 0.001$ significant differences vs. control subjects (derived by the Kruskal–Wallis test). §§ $p < 0.01$ significant differences vs. periodontitis patients. $p < 0.001$.

Moreover, the p-for trend analysis test evidenced that MPO in serum increased gradually in subjects with periodontitis, CVD, and with periodontitis plus CVD (p-trend <0.001) (Figure 3). No statistically significant associations were found in MPO levels between serum and saliva (rs = 0.213, $p = 0.098$). Moreover, in all enrolled patients presented a positive correlation between serum/salivary MPO and hs-CRP levels (rs = 0.341, $p < 0.001$)/(rs = 0.609, $p < 0.001$) (Figure 3).

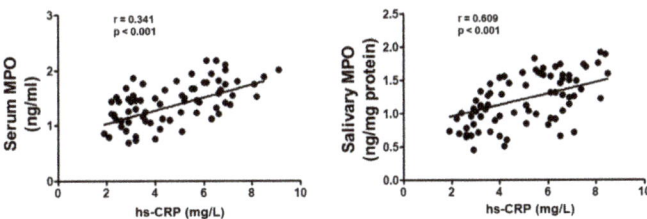

Figure 3. Analysis of correlation of serum and salivary MPO levels with c-reactive protein (CRP) in all patients.

The univariate regression analysis evidenced that there was a significant direct impact of hs-CRP on serum and salivary MPO (both $p < 0.001$). Furthermore, the adjusted multivariate linear regression analysis evidenced that hs-CRP variable was the only significant predictor for serum MPO ($p < 0.001$).

Moreover, hs-CRP ($p < 0.001$) and total cholesterol ($p = 0.035$) were the statistically significant predictor variables for salivary MPO (Table 3).

Table 3. Uni- and multivariate linear regression analysis for MPO levels in serum and saliva in all patients. Age was included as continuous variable. For periodontitis and cardiovascular disease (CVD), controls served as reference. For gender, male served as reference.

Serum MPO Levels		UNIVARIATE			MULTIVARIATE		
	Variable	B	95% CI	p	B	95% CI	p
	CVD	0.442	0.314; 0.558	<0.001	0.122	−0.221; 0.559	0.578
	Periodontitis	0.289	0.18; 0.274	0.024	0.231	−0.066; 0.319	0.226
	hs-CRP	0.278	0.028; 0.136	<0.001	0.314	0.065; 0.189	<0.001
	Age (years)	−0.047	−0.287; 0.056	0.064	−0.039	−0.111; 0.315	0.287
	Female gender	0.212	−0.78; 0.549	0.227	0.219	−0.88; 0.428	0.112
	Education SES	−0.114	−0.178; 0.123	0.287	−0.066	−0.312; 0.398	0.312
Salivary MPO Levels							
	CVD	0.319	0.112; 0.552	<0.001	−0.065	−0.412; 0.289	0.451
	Periodontitis	0.078	−0.069; 0.328	0.411	0.007	−0.178; 0.213	0.665
	hs-CRP	0.082	0.027; 0.287	<0.001	0.066	0.021; 0.133	<0.001
	Age (years)	−0.051	−0.110; 0.036	0.399	0.047	−0.028; 0.087	0.741
	Female gender	0.074	−0.112; 0.211	0.398	0.071	−0.065; 0.412	0.321
	Total Cholesterol	−0.057	−0.151; −0.062	0.037	−0.65	−0.041; 0.314	0.035
	Serum MPO	0.122	−0.021; 0.557	0.057	−0.036	−0.369; 0.166	0.331

4. Discussion

This trial was aimed at evaluating the impact of conditions such as periodontal disease, CVD, or periodontitis plus CVD on MPO levels in serum and saliva. The present trial evidenced that the occurrence of CVD caused increased levels of MPO and hs-CRP in serum and saliva. Nevertheless, in comparison with periodontitis and healthy controls, only the group of subjects with CVD and periodontitis plus CVD had significantly elevated MPO levels in serum and saliva, endorsing the suggestion that CVD influenced the increment of MPO levels in serum and saliva. Furthermore, results of the present study show that the simultaneous presence of periodontitis in patients with CVD can determine an increased activation of MPO and therefore represent a subclinical stimulus for the purpose of an increase in CVD development.

In accordance with the results of the present study, some reports have shown that high levels of MPO in serum represent real independent risk factors of CVD development and increased mortality index, possibly by inactivating NO signaling [33]. Specifically, it has also been shown that, in patients with atherosclerosis, high systemic levels of MPO are associated with significant carotid epithelial dysfunctions, underlining the fundamental inhibitory role of NO exercised by MPO [34].

Therefore, the simultaneous presence of CVD on the one hand and periodontitis on the other hand can be a real explanation for the deterioration of endothelial function due to high levels of MPO. In this regard, recent research has shown that the treatment of periodontitis has significantly reduced the systemic levels of MPO in patients with coronary disease [35].

Moreover, several reports demonstrated that increased hs-CRP levels in serum can facilitate the increment of MPO levels in serum in several diseases in humans [23,35–38]. In accordance with the results of our study, several studies have been demonstrated that situations which may cause an increase of oxidative stress, such as CVD and periodontal disease, cause the high release of CRP, which in turn, can arouse the production of MPO in saliva and serum in order to defend tissue damage determined by oxidative stress condition [36]. In agreement with the results of the present study, Magan-Fernandez et al. [39] demonstrated that CRP and MPO levels were higher during active phases of periodontal disease.

However, while evidence has previously been demonstrated regarding high serum MPO levels as primary mediators of endothelial dysfunction or in the development of cardiovascular risk, from the authors' knowledge, there is no specific evidence to determine MPO levels in saliva in order to evaluate whether the increased expression of salivary MPO levels determines, by reflection, an increase in MPO in serum and then analyzes the salivary levels of MPO as an index of endothelial dysfunction. In this regard, however, it should be noted that this study did not reveal a significant correlation between serum and saliva MPO levels, as salivary MPO levels are influenced in patients enrolled independently only of hs-CRP and total cholesterol. This explanation can be determined by the way that MPO salivary levels may be due to an exclusive local oral production of MPO.

In this regard, it should be noted that, from the studies currently present in the literature, while the effect of MPO at a systemic level mediated by the reduction of NO on endothelial damage has been previously highlighted, the impact of MPO activation orally (e.g., in saliva) is less clear. However, there are studies that show that periodontal disease is positively correlated with high levels of NO and therefore with related stress-oxidative damage [19,24]. The presence of high levels of NO at salivary level can be explained as NO is produced orally in response by the host as a specific salivary defense in the presence of periodontal pathogenic bacteria that are exacerbated during periodontitis [12,24,40]. Furthermore, some studies suggested that decreasing activities of NO and some other enzymatic antioxidants, such as superoxide dismutase catalase, were associated with periodontitis and high levels of MPO, whereas others claim that antioxidants function as protective agents against free radicals during CP progression [19,24,41].

However, there is no unanimous consensus in the literature on the effects of NO levels on tissue damage during periodontitis. Some reports have shown high levels of NO in periodontal tissue in the active periodontal period [39,42] while, on the other hand, other authors have shown lower levels of NO in saliva of subjects with periodontal disease [25,43]. However, results in the literature may have been determined by the different homogeneity of the patients enrolled in the studies, by the different age ranges of the patients analyzed, or by the excessive presence of patients who smoke; in fact it has been shown that smoking can cause a high increase in salivary NO salivary levels [44–46]. Another explanation for the different results found in the literature can be determined by the different salivary sampling method performed in the different studies. Furthermore, the cause of the different expression of MPO at the salivary and serum level may be due to a different production of NO at the oral level which may be different from the serum one.

As an explanation of the results of the present study, it should be highlighted that the dysfunctional damage at the endothelium level found in patients with periodontitis and with CVD can be determined by a specific inflammatory and immune pathway in which MPO modulates a response towards pathogenic bacteria of the oral biofilm which are exacerbated during the active phases of periodontal damage. It has also been shown that MPO, during periodontal disease, mediates the immune response at the endothelial level through specific heat shock proteins which has been shown to be useful for stimulating the production of cross-reactive T cells [47–52]. In this regard, this process which sees

MPO as a key modulator [53–58], has also been shown to influence the host defense mechanism that determines a subsequent activation of endothelial cell production [55,58–63] which leads to an increased risk of future tissue damage effects due to periodontal pathogens bacteria in several oral diseases [43,64–68]. Moreover, the oral microbiota is a key factor in the protection against the colonization of extrinsic pathogens that could impact systemic health [68]. However, the imbalance of the ecosystem together with high levels of MPO, which can be caused by a weak immune system, lead to a challenge for oral and systemic health [68]. The ecological conditions of these habitats are constantly changing, so ecosystems are subject to frequent variations [68,69].

However, the present trial has some limitations. Among the main limitations there is the type of study, which makes it difficult to analyze the cause and effect on a temporal level of MPO. The small sample size, due to high inclusion and exclusion levels, and to the important excluded confounders, also represents a limitation of the present preliminary study. However, the exclusion of several confounders represents a positive and rigorous aspect for the clear evaluation of these confounders on the concentration of serum and salivary levels of MPO.

Recently, different approaches have been developed with the aim of easily evaluating innovative salivary markers useful for early and subclinically validating the development of different diseases. This study indicates that patients suffering from periodontitis and CVD have higher serum and salivary levels of MPO than subjects with periodontitis and healthy subjects.

The results of this study propose that mostly CVD is a stimulus to the increased serum MPO levels which may be beyond a pathway intermediated by hs-CRP. Therefore, these results are promising but at the same time require further studies with a larger sample of analysis in order to better comprehend the function of MPO during periodontitis.

Author Contributions: Conceptualization, A.P.; methodology, S.T.; validation, S.S., formal analysis, M.D.S.; writing—original draft preparation, F.I.; A.L.G. All authors have read and agreed to the published version of the manuscript.

Funding: This research received no external funding.

Conflicts of Interest: The authors declare no conflict of interest.

References

1. Tonetti, M.S.; Greenwell, H.; Kornman, K.S. Staging and grading of periodontitis: Framework and proposal of a new classification and case definition. *J. Periodontol.* **2018**, *89* (Suppl. 1), S159–S172. [CrossRef] [PubMed]
2. Briguglio, F.; Briguglio, E.; Briguglio, R.; Cafiero, C.; Isola, G. Treatment of infrabony periodontal defects using a resorbable biopolymer of hyaluronic acid: a randomized clinical trial. *Quintessence Int.* **2013**, *44*, 231–240. [PubMed]
3. Eke, P.I.; Wei, L.; Thornton-Evans, G.O.; Borrell, L.N.; Borgnakke, W.S.; Dye, B.; Genco, R.J. Risk Indicators for Periodontitis in US Adults: NHANES 2009 to 2012. *J. Periodontol.* **2016**, *87*, 1174–1185. [CrossRef] [PubMed]
4. Isola, G.; Alibrandi, A.; Currò, M.; Matarese, M.; Ricca, S.; Matarese, G.; Ientile, R.; Kocher, T. Evaluation of salivary and serum ADMA levels in patients with periodontal and cardiovascular disease as subclinical marker of cardiovascular risk. *J. Periodontol.* **2020**. [CrossRef]
5. Isola, G.; Giudice, A.L.; Polizzi, A.; Alibrandi, A.; Patini, R.; Ferlito, S. Periodontitis and Tooth Loss Have Negative Systemic Impact on Circulating Progenitor Cell Levels: a Clinical Study. *Genes* **2019**, *10*, 1022. [CrossRef]
6. Holmlund, A.; Holm, G.; Lind, L. Number of Teeth as a Predictor of Cardiovascular Mortality in a Cohort of 7,674 Subjects Followed for 12 Years. *J. Periodontol.* **2010**, *81*, 870–876. [CrossRef]
7. Isola, G.; Polizzi, A.; Alibrandi, A.; Indelicato, F.; Ferlito, S. Analysis of Endothelin-1 concentrations in individuals with periodontitis. *Sci. Rep.* **2020**. [CrossRef]
8. Li, C.; Lv, Z.; Shi, Z.; Zhu, Y.; Wu, Y.; Li, L.; Iheozor-Ejiofor, Z. Periodontal therapy for the management of cardiovascular disease in patients with chronic periodontitis. *Cochrane Database Syst. Rev.* **2017**, *2017*, CD009197. [CrossRef]
9. Isola, G.; Polizzi, A.; Muraglie, S.; Leonardi, R.; Giudice, A.L. Assessment of Vitamin C and Antioxidant Profiles in Saliva and Serum in Patients with Periodontitis and Ischemic Heart Disease. *Nutrients* **2019**, *11*, 2956. [CrossRef]

10. Matarese, G.; Curro, M.; Isola, G.; Caccamo, D.; Vecchio, M.; Giunta, M.L.; Ramaglia, L.; Cordasco, G.; Williams, R.C.; Ientile, R. Transglutaminase 2 up-regulation is associated with RANKL/OPG pathway in cultured HPDL cells and THP-1-differentiated macrophages. *Amino Acids* **2015**, *47*, 2447–2455. [CrossRef]
11. Aratani, Y. Myeloperoxidase: Its role for host defense, inflammation, and neutrophil function. *Arch. Biochem. Biophys.* **2018**, *640*, 47–52. [CrossRef] [PubMed]
12. Ahmad, S.; Ramadori, G.; Moriconi, F. Modulation of Chemokine- and Adhesion-Molecule Gene Expression and Recruitment of Neutrophil Granulocytes in Rat and Mouse Liver after a Single Gadolinium Chloride or Zymosan Treatment. *Int. J. Mol. Sci.* **2018**, *19*, 3891. [CrossRef] [PubMed]
13. de Souza, R.G.M.; Gomes, A.C.; Navarro, A.M.; Cunha, L.C.D.; Silva, M.A.C.; Junior, F.B.; Mota, J.F. Baru Almonds Increase the Activity of Glutathione Peroxidase in Overweight and Obese Women: a Randomized, Placebo-Controlled Trial. *Nutrients* **2019**, *11*, 1750. [CrossRef] [PubMed]
14. Isola, G.; Matarese, G.; Giudice, G.L.; Briguglio, F.; Alibrandi, A.; Crupi, A.; Cordasco, G.; Ramaglia, L. a New Approach for the Treatment of Lateral Periodontal Cysts with an 810-nm Diode Laser. *Int. J. Periodontics Restor. Dent.* **2017**, *37*, 120–129. [CrossRef] [PubMed]
15. Matarese, G.; Isola, G.; Anastasi, G.P.; Cutroneo, G.; Favaloro, A.; Vita, G.; Cordasco, G.; Milardi, D.; Zizzari, V.L.; Tetè, S.; et al. Transforming Growth Factor Beta 1 and Vascular Endothelial Growth Factor levels in the pathogenesis of periodontal disease. *Eur. J. Inflamm.* **2013**, *11*, 479–488. [CrossRef]
16. Peniche-Palma, D.C.; Carrillo-Avila, B.A.; Sauri-Esquivel, E.A.; Acosta-Viana, K.; Esparza-Villalpando, V.; Pozos-Guillen, A.; Hernandez-Rios, M.; Martinez-Aguilar, V.M. Levels of Myeloperoxidase and Metalloproteinase-9 in Gingival Crevicular Fluid from Diabetic Subjects with and without Stage 2, Grade B Periodontitis. *BioMed Res. Int.* **2019**, *2019*, 5613514. [CrossRef]
17. Currò, M.; Matarese, G.; Isola, G.; Caccamo, D.; Ventura, V.P.; Cornelius, C.; Lentini, M.; Cordasco, G.; Ientile, R. Differential expression of transglutaminase genes in patients with chronic periodontitis. *Oral Dis.* **2014**, *20*, 616–623. [CrossRef]
18. Isola, G.; Williams, R.C.; Lo Gullo, A.; Ramaglia, L.; Matarese, M.; Iorio-Siciliano, V.; Cosio, C.; Matarese, G. Risk association between scleroderma disease characteristics, periodontitis, and tooth loss. *Clin Rheumatol.* **2017**, *36*, 2733–2741. [CrossRef]
19. Andrukhov, O.; Haririan, H.; Bertl, K.; Rausch, W.-D.; Bantleon, H.-P.; Moritz, A.; Rausch-Fan, X. Nitric oxide production, systemic inflammation and lipid metabolism in periodontitis patients: Possible gender aspect. *J. Clin. Periodontol.* **2013**, *40*, 916–923. [CrossRef]
20. Isola, G.; Alibrandi, A.; Rapisarda, E.; Matarese, G.; Williams, R.C.; Leonardi, R. Association of vitamin d in patients with periodontitis: a cross-sectional study. *J. Periodontal Res.* **2020**, in press.
21. Gurav, A.N. The implication of periodontitis in vascular endothelial dysfunction. *Eur. J. Clin. Investig.* **2014**, *44*, 1000–1009. [CrossRef]
22. Tabeta, K.; Hosojima, M.; Nakajima, M.; Miyauchi, S.; Miyazawa, H.; Takahashi, N.; Matsuda, Y.; Sugita, N.; Komatsu, Y.; Sato, K.; et al. Increased serum PCSK9, a potential biomarker to screen for periodontitis, and decreased total bilirubin associated with probing depth in a Japanese community survey. *J. Periodontal Res.* **2018**, *53*, 446–456. [CrossRef]
23. Isola, G.; Ramaglia, L.; Cordasco, G.; Lucchese, A.; Fiorillo, L.; Matarese, G. The effect of a functional appliance in the management of temporomandibular joint disorders in patients with juvenile idiopathic arthritis. *Minerva Stomatol.* **2017**, *66*, 1–8. [PubMed]
24. Kendall, H.K.; Marshall, R.I.; Bartold, P.M. Nitric oxide, and tissue destruction. *Oral Dis.* **2001**, *7*, 2–10. [CrossRef] [PubMed]
25. Aurer, A.; Aleksic, J.; Ivic-Kardum, M.; Aurer, J.; Čulo, F. Nitric oxide synthesis is decreased in periodontitis. *J. Clin. Periodontol.* **2001**, *28*, 565–568. [CrossRef] [PubMed]
26. Ruest, L.B.; Ranjbaran, H.; Tong, E.J.; Svoboda, K.K.H.; Feng, J.Q. Activation of Receptor Activator of Nuclear Factor-κB Ligand and Matrix Metalloproteinase Production in Periodontal Fibroblasts by Endothelin Signaling. *J. Periodontol.* **2016**, *87*, e1–e8. [CrossRef] [PubMed]
27. von Elm, E.; Altman, D.G.; Egger, M.; Pocock, S.J.; Gotzsche, P.C.; Vandenbroucke, J.P. The Strengthening the Reporting of Observational Studies in Epidemiology (STROBE) statement: Guidelines for reporting observational studies. *J. Clin. Periodontol.* **2008**, *61*, 344–349. [CrossRef]
28. Lindhe, J.; Ranney, R.; Lamster, I.; Charles, A.; Chung, C.-P.; Flemmig, T.; Kinane, D.; Listgarten, M.; Löe, H.; Schoor, R.; et al. Consensus Report: Chronic Periodontitis. *Ann. Periodontol.* **1999**, *4*, 38. [CrossRef]

29. Isola, G.; Matarese, M.; Ramaglia, L.; Iorio-Siciliano, V.; Cordasco, G.; Matarese, G. Efficacy of a drug composed of herbal extracts on postoperative discomfort after surgical removal of impacted mandibular third molar: a randomized, triple-blind, controlled clinical trial. *Clin. Oral Investig.* **2019**, *23*, 2443–2453. [CrossRef]
30. Bassand, J.P.; Hamm, C.W.; Ardissino, D.; Boersma, E.; Budaj, A.; Fernández-Avilés, F.; Fox, K.A.; Hasdai, D.; Ohman, E.M.; Wallentin, L.; et al. Guidelines for the diagnosis and treatment of non-ST-segment elevation acute coronary syndromes: The Task Force for the Diagnosis and Treatment of Non-ST-Segment Elevation Acute Coronary Syndromes of the European Society of Cardiology. *Eur. Heart J.* **2007**, *28*, 1598–1660. [CrossRef]
31. O'Leary, T.J.; Drake, R.B.; Naylor, J.E. The Plaque Control Record. *J. Periodontol.* **1972**, *43*, 38. [CrossRef] [PubMed]
32. Hollander, M.; Wolfe, D.A.; Chicken, E. *Nonparametric Statistical Methods*, 3rd ed.; John Wiley & Sons: Hoboken, NJ, USA, 2013.
33. Lo Giudice, G.; Lo Giudice, R.; Matarese, G.; Isola, G.; Cicciù, M.; Terranova, A.; Palaia, G.; Romeo, U. Evaluation of magnification systems in restorative dentistry. An in-vitro study. *Dental Cadmos* **2015**, *83*, 296–305. [CrossRef]
34. Mazzoli, A.; Crescenzo, R.; Cigliano, L.; Spagnuolo, M.S.; Cancelliere, R.; Gatto, C.; Iossa, S. Early Hepatic Oxidative Stress and Mitochondrial Changes Following Western Diet in Middle Aged Rats. *Nutrients* **2019**, *11*, 2670. [CrossRef]
35. Lahdentausta, L.; Paju, S.; Mäntylä, P.; Buhlin, K.; Pietiäinen, M.; Tervahartiala, T.; Nieminen, M.S.; Sinisalo, J.; Sorsa, T.; Pussinen, P.J. Smoking confounds the periodontal diagnostics using saliva biomarkers. *J. Periodontol.* **2019**, *90*, 475–483. [CrossRef]
36. Isola, G.; Matarese, G.; Ramaglia, L.; Pedullà, E.; Rapisarda, E.; Iorio-Siciliano, V. Association between periodontitis and glycosylated haemoglobin before diabetes onset: a cross-sectional study. *Clin. Oral Investig.* **2019**. [CrossRef]
37. Valenzuela, M.; Draibe, J.; Quero, M.; Fulladosa, X.; Cruzado, J.M.; Bestard, O.; Torras, J.; Valenzuela, L.M. Exploring Frequencies of Circulating Specific Th17 Cells against Myeloperoxidase and Proteinase 3 in ANCA Associated Vasculitis. *Int. J. Mol. Sci.* **2019**, *20*, 5820. [CrossRef]
38. Przepiera-Będzak, H.; Fischer, K.; Brzosko, M. Serum Interleukin-18, Fetuin-A, Soluble Intercellular Adhesion Molecule-1, and Endothelin-1 in Ankylosing Spondylitis, Psoriatic Arthritis, and SAPHO Syndrome. *Int. J. Mol. Sci.* **2016**, *17*, 1255. [CrossRef]
39. Magán-Fernández, A.; O'Valle, F.; Abadía-Molina, F.; Muñoz, R.; Puga-Guil, P.; Mesa, F. Characterization and comparison of neutrophil extracellular traps in gingival samples of periodontitis and gingivitis: a pilot study. *J. Periodontal Res.* **2019**, *54*, 218–224. [CrossRef]
40. Cavuoti, S.; Matarese, G.; Isola, G.; Abdolreza, J.; Femiano, F.; Perillo, L. Combined orthodontic-surgical management of a transmigrated mandibular canine: a case report. *Angle Orthod.* **2016**, *86*, 681–691. [CrossRef]
41. Matejka, M.; Partyka, L.; Ulm, C.; Solar, P.; Sinzinger, H. Nitric oxide synthesis is increased in periodontal disease. *J. Periodontal Res.* **1998**, *33*, 517–518. [CrossRef]
42. Perillo, L.; Isola, G.; Esercizio, D.; Iovane, M.; Triolo, G.; Matarese, G. Differences in craniofacial characteristics in Southern Italian children from Naples: a retrospective study by cephalometric analysis. *Eur. J. Paediatr. Dent.* **2013**, *14*, 195–198. [PubMed]
43. Ozer, L.; Elgün, S.; Özdemir, B.; Pervane, B.; Özmeriç, N. Arginine–Nitric Oxide–Polyamine Metabolism in Periodontal Disease. *J. Periodontol.* **2011**, *82*, 320–328. [CrossRef]
44. Bodis, S.; Haregewoin, A. Significantly reduced salivary nitric oxide levels in smokers. *Ann. Oncol.* **1994**, *5*, 371–372. [CrossRef]
45. Vasconcelos, D.F.P.; Da Silva, F.R.P.; Pinto, M.E.S.C.; Santana, L.D.A.B.; Souza, I.G.; De Souza, L.K.M.; Oliveira, N.C.M.; Ventura, C.A.; Novaes, P.D.; Barbosa, A.L.D.R.; et al. Decrease of Pericytes is Associated with Liver Disease Caused by Ligature-Induced Periodontitis in Rats. *J. Periodontol.* **2017**, *88*, e49–e57. [CrossRef] [PubMed]
46. Isola, G.; Polizzi, A.; Santonocito, S.; Alibrandi, A.; Ferlito, S. Expression of Salivary and Serum Malondialdehyde and Lipid Profile of Patients with Periodontitis and Coronary Heart Disease. *Int. J. Mol. Sci.* **2019**, *20*, 6061. [CrossRef] [PubMed]
47. Isola, G.; Matarese, M.; Ramaglia, L.; Cicciù, M.; Matarese, G. Evaluation of the efficacy of celecoxib and ibuprofen on postoperative pain, swelling, and mouth opening after surgical removal of impacted third

molars: a randomized, controlled clinical trial. *Int. J. Oral Maxillofac. Surg.* **2019**, *48*, 1348–1354. [CrossRef] [PubMed]

48. Isola, G.; Perillo, L.; Migliorati, M.; Matarese, M.; Dalessandri, D.; Grassia, V.; Alibrandi, A.; Matarese, G. The impact of temporomandibular joint arthritis on functional disability and global health in patients with juvenile idiopathic arthritis. *Eur. J. Orthod.* **2019**, *41*, 117–124. [CrossRef]

49. Isola, G.; Anastasi, G.P.; Matarese, G.; Williams, R.C.; Cutroneo, G.; Bracco, P.; Piancino, M.G. Functional and molecular outcomes of the human masticatory muscles. *Oral Dis.* **2018**, *24*, 1428–1441. [CrossRef]

50. Isola, G.; Alibrandi, A.; Pedullà, E.; Grassia, V.; Ferlito, S.; Perillo, L.; Rapisarda, E. Analysis of the Effectiveness of Lornoxicam and Flurbiprofen on Management of Pain and Sequelae Following Third Molar Surgery: a Randomized, Controlled, Clinical Trial. *J. Clin. Med.* **2019**, *8*, 325. [CrossRef]

51. Camacho-Alonso, F.; Davia-Peña, R.S.; Vilaplana-Vivo, C.; Tudela-Mulero, M.R.; Merino, J.J.; Martínez-Beneyto, Y. Synergistic effect of photodynamic therapy and alendronate on alveolar bone loss in rats with ligature-induced periodontitis. *J. Periodontal Res.* **2017**, *53*, 306–314. [CrossRef]

52. Isola, G.; Matarese, G.; Alibrandi, A.; Dalessandri, D.; Migliorati, M.; Pedullà, E.; Rapisarda, E. Comparison of Effectiveness of Etoricoxib and Diclofenac on Pain and Perioperative Sequelae After Surgical Avulsion of Mandibular Third Molars: a Randomized, Controlled, Clinical Trial. *Clin. J. Pain* **2019**, *35*, 908–915. [CrossRef]

53. Mohammed, H.; Varoni, E.M.; Cochis, A.; Cordaro, M.; Gallenzi, P.; Patini, R.; Staderini, E.; Lajolo, C.; Rimondini, L.; Rocchetti, V. Oral Dysbiosis in Pancreatic Cancer and Liver Cirrhosis: a Review of the Literature. *Biomedicines* **2018**, *6*, 115. [CrossRef] [PubMed]

54. Patini, R.; Gallenzi, P.; Spagnuolo, G.; Cordaro, M.; Cantiani, M.; Amalfitano, A.; Arcovito, A.; Callà, C.; Mingrone, G.; Nocca, G. Correlation Between Metabolic Syndrome, Periodontitis and Reactive Oxygen Species Production. a Pilot Study. *Open Dent. J.* **2017**, *11*, 621–627. [CrossRef]

55. Caccianiga, G.; Paiusco, A.; Perillo, L.; Nucera, R.; Pinsino, A.; Maddalone, M.; Cordasco, G.; Giudice, A.L. Does Low-Level Laser Therapy Enhance the Efficiency of Orthodontic Dental Alignment? Results from a Randomized Pilot Study. *Photomed. Laser Surg.* **2017**, *35*, 421–426. [CrossRef] [PubMed]

56. Lo Giudice, A.; Nucera, R.; Leonardi, R.; Paiusco, A.; Baldoni, M.; Caccianiga, G. a Comparative Assessment of the Efficiency of Orthodontic Treatment with and Without Photobiomodulation during Mandibular Decrowding in Young Subjects: a Single-Center, Single-Blind Randomized Controlled Trial. *Photobiomodul. Photomed. Laser Surg.* **2020**. [CrossRef]

57. Ferlazzo, N.; Currò, M.; Zinellu, A.; Caccamo, D.; Isola, G.; Ventura, V.; Carru, C.; Matarese, G.; Ientile, R. Influence of MTHFR genetic background on P16 and MGMT methylation in oral squamous cell cancer. *Int. J. Mol. Sci.* **2017**, *18*, 724. [CrossRef]

58. Cutroneo, G.; Piancino, M.G.; Ramieri, G.; Bracco, P.; Vita, G.; Isola, G.; Vermiglio, G.; Favaloro, A.; Anastasi, G.P.; Trimarchi, F. Expression of muscle-specific integrins in masseter muscle fibers during malocclusion disease. *Int. J. Mol. Med.* **2012**, *30*, 235–242. [CrossRef]

59. Isola, G.; Matarese, M.; Briguglio, F.; Grassia, V.; Picciolo, G.; Fiorillo, L.; Matarese, G. Effectiveness of Low-Level Laser Therapy during Tooth Movement: a Randomized Clinical Trial. *Materials* **2019**, *12*, 2187. [CrossRef]

60. Piancino, M.G.; Isola, G.; Cannavale, R.; Cutroneo, G.; Vermiglio, G.; Bracco, P.; Anastasi, G.P.; Grazia, P.M.; Gaetano, I.; Rosangela, C.; et al. From periodontal mechanoreceptors to chewing motor control: a systematic review. *Arch. Oral Boil.* **2017**, *78*, 109–121. [CrossRef]

61. Lo Giudice, A.; Nucera, R.; Perillo, L.; Paiusco, A.; Caccianiga, G. Is low-level laser therapy an effective method to alleviate pain induced by active orthodontic alignment archwire? a randomized clinical trial. *J. Evid. Based Dent. Pract.* **2019**, *19*, 71–78. [CrossRef]

62. Leonardi, R.; Lo Giudice, A.; Rugeri, M.; Muraglie, S.; Cordasco, G.; Barbato, E. Three-dimensional evaluation on digital casts of maxillary palatal size and morphology in patients with functional posterior crossbite. *Eur. J. Orthod.* **2018**, *40*, 556–562. [CrossRef] [PubMed]

63. Giudice, A.L.; Caccianiga, G.; Crimi, S.; Cavallini, C.; Leonardi, R. Frequency and type of ponticulus posticus in a longitudinal sample of nonorthodontically treated patients: Relationship with gender, age, skeletal maturity, and skeletal malocclusion. *Oral Surg. Oral Med. Oral Pathol. Oral Radiol.* **2018**, *126*, 291–297. [CrossRef] [PubMed]
64. Cannavale, R.; Matarese, G.; Isola, G.; Grassia, V.; Perillo, L. Early treatment of an ectopic premolar to prevent molar-premolar transposition. *Am. J. Orthod. Dentofacial Orthop.* **2013**, *143*, 559–569. [CrossRef] [PubMed]
65. Matarese, G.; Isola, G.; Alibrandi, A.; Lo Gullo, A.; Bagnato, G.; Cordasco, G.; Perillo, L. Occlusal and MRI characterizations in systemic sclerosis patients: a prospective study from Southern Italian cohort. *Joint. Bone. Spine.* **2016**, *83*, 57–62. [CrossRef] [PubMed]
66. Isola, G.; Matarese, G.; Cordasco, G.; Rotondo, F.; Crupi, A.; Ramaglia, L. Anticoagulant therapy in patients undergoing dental interventions: a critical review of the literature and current perspectives. *Minerva Stomatol.* **2015**, *64*, 21–46. [PubMed]
67. Matarese, G.; Isola, G.; Ramaglia, L.; Dalessandri, D.; Lucchese, A.; Alibrandi, A.; Fabiano, F.; Cordasco, G. Periodontal biotype: characteristic, prevalence and dimensions related to dental malocclusion. *Minerva Stomatol.* **2016**, *65*, 231–238.
68. Bourgeois, D.; Inquimbert, C.; Ottolenghi, L.; Carrouel, F. Periodontal Pathogens as Risk Factors of Cardiovascular Diseases, Diabetes, Rheumatoid Arthritis, Cancer, and Chronic Obstructive Pulmonary Disease-Is There Cause for Consideration? *Microorganisms* **2019**, *7*, 424. [CrossRef]
69. Khan, A.A.; Alsahli, M.A.; Rahmani, A.H. Myeloperoxidase as an Active Disease Biomarker: Recent Biochemical and Pathological Perspectives. *Med. Sci.* **2018**, *6*, 33. [CrossRef]

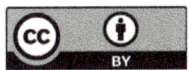

© 2020 by the authors. Licensee MDPI, Basel, Switzerland. This article is an open access article distributed under the terms and conditions of the Creative Commons Attribution (CC BY) license (http://creativecommons.org/licenses/by/4.0/).

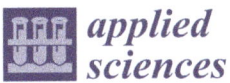

Review

The Efficacy of Retention Appliances after Fixed Orthodontic Treatment: A Systematic Review and Meta-Analysis

Antonino Lo Giudice [1], Gaetano Isola [2,*], Lorenzo Rustico [3], Vincenzo Ronsivalle [1], Marco Portelli [3] and Riccardo Nucera [3,*]

1. Department of Medical-Surgical Specialties—Section of Orthodontics, School of Dentistry, University of Catania, Policlinico Universitario "G. Rodolico" Via Santa Sofia 78, 95123 Catania, Italy; nino.logiudice@gmail.com (A.L.G.); vincenzo.ronsivalle@hotmail.it (V.R.)
2. Department of Medical-Surgical Specialties, School of Dentistry, University of Catania, Policlinico Universitario "G. Rodolico" Via Santa Sofia 78, 95123 Catania, Italy
3. Department of Biomedical and Dental Sciences and Morphofunctional Imaging, Section of Orthodontics, School of Dentistry, University of Messina, Policlinico Universitario "G. Martino," 98100 Messina, Italy; lorenzo.rustico@gmail.com (L.R.); mportelli@unime.it (M.P.)
* Correspondence: gaetano.isola@unict.it (G.I.); riccardo.nucera@gmail.com (R.N.); Tel.: +39-095-3782453 (G.I.)

Received: 26 March 2020; Accepted: 26 April 2020; Published: 29 April 2020

Abstract: The purpose of this article is to evaluate the amount of the relapse of anterior crowding and the efficacy of retention appliances by reviewing the best available scientific evidence. A survey of articles published up to November 2019 about the stability of dental alignment and retention after fixed orthodontic treatment was performed using seven electronic databases. Study Selection: Only randomized clinical trials investigating patients previously treated with multi-bracket appliances with a follow-up period longer than 6 months were included. Data Extraction: Two authors independently performed the study selection, data extraction, and risk of bias assessment. All pooled data analyses were performed using a random-effects model. Statistical heterogeneity was evaluated. In total, eight randomized clinical trials (RCTs) were included, grouping data from 987 patients. The ages of the patients varied across the studies, ranging between 13 and 17 years. The observation period ranged between 6 and 24 months. The data showed no significant intercanine width modifications during the retention period with both fixed and removable retainers. A significant modification of Little's Index was found for the mandibular removable retainers with a mean difference of 0.72 mm (95% Cl, 0.47 to 0.98) and for the maxillary removable retainers with a mean difference of 0.48 mm (95% Cl, 0.27 to 0.68). No significant changes were found by evaluating Little's Index modification for the mandibular fixed retainers. The results of this meta-analysis showed that all the considered retainers were effective in maintaining dental alignment after fixed orthodontic treatment. However, fixed retainers showed greater efficacy compared to removable retainers.

Keywords: relapse; orthodontic retainers; stability; systematic review; meta-analysis

1. Introduction

Stable tooth position after orthodontic treatment is considered a treatment goal. However, evidence shows that the majority of orthodontic treatments move teeth from a stable to an unstable position [1]. In this way, the use of a retainer is considered the only method able to maintain occlusal results [2]. Post-treatment tooth stability can be affected by several different factors, including bone and soft tissue development [3], primary crowding [4–6], dental eruption [7], modification of arch form [8], post-treatment occlusion [9], and the characteristics of pre-treatment malocclusion [10]. Retention can be performed by placing removable or fixed retainers. A recent Cochrane review reported a lack of evidence concerning the effectiveness different retention methods [11]. The efficacy of different retention appliances is of great interest for clinicians to support clinical retention protocols [12–14]. The literature does not provide meta-analytic data reporting and comparing the amount of relapse that occurs when using different retention appliances. The aim of this systematic review and meta-analysis was to evaluate the amount of relapse of anterior crowding and consequently to evaluate the efficacy of retention appliances used after fixed orthodontic treatment according to the best scientific evidence available [15].

2. Materials and Methods

The present systematic review with meta-analysis was performed according to the guidelines provided by the Cochrane Handbook for Systematic Reviews of Interventions (version 5.1.0) and was reported according to the PRISMA statement [16–19]. The protocol of this meta-analysis was preliminary registered on PROSPERO (https://www.crd.york.ac.uk/prospero/). Two authors independently carried out the selection of the studies, data collection, and the assessment of the risk of bias. Any disagreement was resolved by discussion with a third author. The level of agreement between the 2 reviewers was assessed by Cohen kappa statistics, for which a threshold value of 0.90 was preset.

2.1. Information Sources and Search

A survey of articles published up to November 2019 on stability and retention after orthodontic treatment was performed using several electronic databases (Table 1).

Table 1. Performed electronic searches.

Database of Published Trials	Search Strategy Used	Hits
MEDLINE searched via PubMed searched on November 18, 2019 via www.ncbi.nlm.nih.gov/sites/entrez/	(((((incisor stability [tiab]) OR post treatment stability [tiab]) OR relapse [mesh])) AND ((((orthodontic treatment [tiab] or Orthodontic fixed appliance [tiab]) Or orthodontic retainer [tiab])	254
OvidSP searched on November 18, 2019 via https://ovidsp.tx.ovid.com	(incisor stability OR post treatment stability OR relapse) AND (orthodontic treatment OR orthodontic fixed appliance OR orthodontic retainers)	1135
EMBASE searched via ScienceDirect searched on November 18, 2019 via www.embase.com	(incisor stability or post treatment stability or relapse) AND (orthodontic treatment or orthodontic fixed appliance or orthodontic retainers)	1174
Cochrane Database of Systematic Reviews searched via The Cochrane Library searched on November 18, 2019 via www.thecochranelibrary.com	(incisor stability OR post treatment stability OR relapse) AND (orthodontic treatment OR orthodontic fixed appliance OR orthodontic retainers)	2
Cochrane Central Register of Controlled Trials searched via The Cochrane Library searched on January 18, 2018 via www.thecochranelibrary.com	(incisor stability OR post treatment stability OR relapse) AND (orthodontic treatment OR orthodontic fixed appliance OR orthodontic retainers)	94
Scopus searched on November 18, 2019 via www.scopus.com	(incisor stability OR post treatment stability OR relapse) AND (orthodontic treatment OR orthodontic fixed appliance OR orthodontic retainers)	191
Web of Science searched on November 18, 2019 via http://scientific.thomson.com/products/wos	(incisor stability or post treatment stability or relapse) AND (orthodontic treatment or orthodontic fixed appliance or orthodontic retainers)	745
Total		3595

Previous systematic reviews and meta-analyses on this topic were also identified, and their reference lists were scanned to find additional trials. No restriction was applied to language, publication year, or status.

2.2. Selection of Studies

Duplicated reports were preliminary excluded. All retrieved records were screened on the basis of their titles and abstracts, and the full texts of the remaining articles were assessed for eligibility in the final analysis.

Studies were considered eligible if they met the following criteria (reported according to the PICO format): clinical trials on human subjects, orthodontic patients treated with multi-bracket appliances with no craniofacial deformity (population), orthodontic retention performed with fixed or removable retainers (intervention), a comparable control group (control group), results analyzed at the beginning of retention and after a follow-up period longer than 6 months (outcomes measured), and analyzed treatment effects that were not influenced by concomitant and/or additional therapeutic procedures.

2.3. Data Extraction and Management

A data extraction form was developed to collect the characteristics (study design, type of retention appliance, sample size, age, sex, orthodontic treatment characteristics, setting, observation time, type of measurements, and follow-up) and outcomes from the included studies. Relapse after orthodontic treatment was investigated by using two parameters: Little's Irregularity Index (LII) for assessment of the degree of crowding and intercanine width for assessment of the transversal anterior dental arch width.

2.4. Assessment of Risk of Bias

The risk of bias assessment was performed using the Cochrane Collaboration's risk of bias tool (Review Manager version 5.2; Nordic Cochrane Centre, Cochrane Collaboration, Copenhagen, Denmark, 2012). Each randomized clinical trial (RCT) was assigned an overall risk of bias rating: low risk (low for all key domains), high risk (high for ≥1 key domain), or unclear risk (unclear for ≥1 key domain).

2.5. Summary Measures and Data Analysis

Two outcomes were considered for the meta-analytic analysis: Little's Irregularity Index and Intercanine width. The published clinical trials evaluating retention protocols do not have a control group with un-retained patients for ethical reasons. As a consequence, all the published trials compare two or more treatment protocols. In order to obtain a quantitative estimation of occlusal changes occurred with different retention protocols, we considered the single-arm data of clinical trials as the data obtained from case-series studies, and we performed a meta-analysis extrapolating and combining these data. In terms of data characteristics, the single-arm data from the RCTs and case series studies data are equivalent, as both studies report data with a mean value and standard deviation. However, the data extrapolated from the single-arm RCTs present less bias compared to the data from the case series studies. Finally, our strategy was supported by the literature. Indeed, when clinical trials with untreated control groups are not available, case-series studies without a control group can be used to perform a meta-analysis [20–22].

The considered effects size used for the meta-analysis was the difference between the outcome values at the end of treatment with fixed appliances and the outcome values after the retention period. Some studies reported the interquartile range rather than standard deviation, and the data extracted from those studies were properly adjusted [23]. The mean differences (MDs) and their corresponding 95% confidence intervals (95% CIs) were used to summarize and combine the data. A random-effects model was applied to estimate all the pooled data. This analysis was performed by means of the OpenMeta [Analyst] computer program (http://www.cebm.brown.edu/openmeta/) [24]. A third outcome (i.e., the fixed retainer failure rate) was considered only for qualitative evaluation.

2.6. Assessment of Heterogeneity

Clinical heterogeneity was evaluated by examining the types of participants and the interventions for the outcome in each included study. For all analyses, heterogeneity was assessed with the I^2 index, which is an indicator of true heterogeneity in percentages [14–19].

2.7. Assessment of Quality of Evidence

The quality of evidence was assessed using the Grades of Recommendation, Assessment, Development, and Evaluation Pro software (GRADEPro) [25]. The strength of the recommendation for each outcome investigated was assessed using the Strength of Recommendation Taxonomy (SORT) Grading system [26], which addresses the issue of patient-oriented (effectiveness) versus disease-oriented evidence (efficacy). POEMs (patient oriented evidence that matters) allows clinicians to filter information from the medical literature and focus only on what is in fact important for the patient [26].

2.8. Sensitivity Analysis

A sensitivity analysis was conducted to evaluate the LII modification in the lower arch with the mandibular removable retention appliances, excluding the RCT with the highest risk of bias (Figure S1).

3. Results

3.1. This Study Selection

Figure 1 shows the flow diagram for the selection of studies. Supplementary Table S1 reports the number of excluded studies and the reasons for exclusion. Eleven studies [21–31] were selected for the qualitative analysis and eight studies for the final quantitative synthesis [21–28] (Table 1). The inter-reviewer agreements for study selection were suitable, with a kappa value of 0.987.

3.2. Study Characteristics

The characteristics of the 11 RCTs included for the qualitative synthesis are summarized in Table 2. All eight RCTs selected for the meta-analysis evaluated the efficacy of different type of retention appliances (both removable and fixed) after orthodontic treatment with a multi-bracket appliance; the majority of trials took place in university settings. The total number of pooled observed patients was 987. Six studies [27,30–34] included both male and female participants, while in two studies [28,31], the authors did not specify the numbers of male and female participants. Five studies [27,29,30,33,34] reported the patients' ages, with an age range between 13 and 17 years. The appliance features were heterogeneous among the selected studies: Six trials evaluated the effects of vacuum-formed retainers [27,30–34], four trials evaluated the effects of bonded fixed retainers [27–31], two trials evaluated the effects of a Hawley retainer [33,34], one trial evaluated the effects of a Begg retainer [31], and one trial evaluated the effects of a positioner [27].

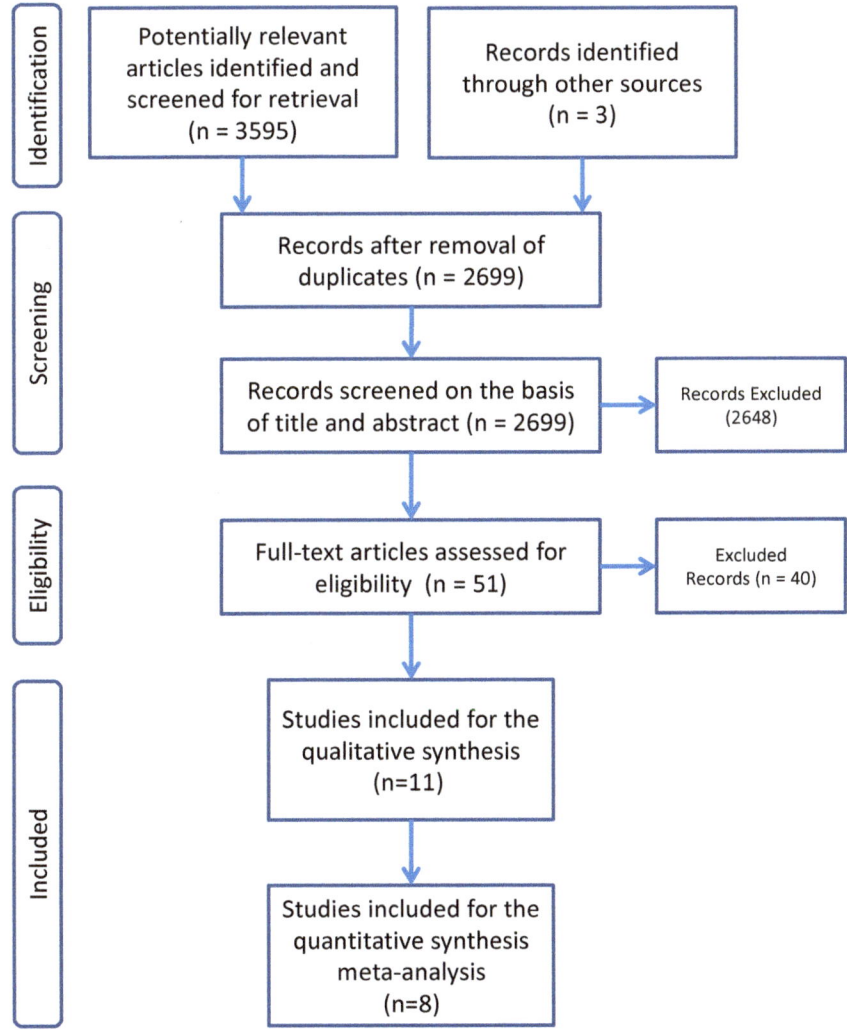

Figure 1. Flow Chart.

Seven studies [27,29,30,32–34] reported the percentage of patients treated with or without extraction, as shown in Table 2. The times of daily wear for the removable appliances (vacuum-formed retainers, Hawley retainers, Begg retainers, and positioners) varied between full-time and night-time among the RCTs, and the observation time varied from 6 to 24 months. The inter-reviewer agreements for study selection were suitable, with a kappa value of 0.968.

Table 2. Study characteristics.

Selected References	Maxillary Retention	Mandibular Retention	Sample	Sex	Age (y)	Orthodontic Treatment Characteristics	Setting	Observation Time	Methods of Measurement
Bolla et al. (2012)	Fixed Retainer (GFR) Fixed Retainer (MST)	Fixed Retainer (GFR) Fixed Retainer (MST)	GFR = 40 MST = 45	F = 28 M = 12 F = 28 M = 17	F = 20.2 M = 23.4 F = 22.6 M = 24.1	No Extraction: 100% Extraction: 0%	Italy	6 years	Failure rate.
Edman Tynelius et al. (2013)	Vacum-Formed Retainer Positioner	Fixed Retainer Positioner	VFR = 47 Positioner = 22 FR = 24	F = 45 M = 30	14,4	No Extraction: 0% Extraction: 100%	National Health Service (NHS) Ystad, Sweden	24 months	Little's irregularity index (LII), intercanine width.
Egli et al. (2017)	//	Fixed Retainer (DB) Fixed Retainer (IB)	FR (DB) = 30 FR (IB) = 30	//	//	//	Postgraduate orthodontic clinic University of Geneva, Switzerland.	24 months	Intercanine width, failure rate.
Forde et al. (2017)	Bonded Retainer Vacum-Formed Retainer	Bonded Retainer Vacum-Formed Retainer	BR = 30 VFR = 26	F = 15 M = 15 F = 18 F = 12	BR = 16 VFR = 17	No Extraction: 31,6% Extraction: 68,4%	St Luke's Hospital, Bradford and York Hospital and Leeds Dental Institute; UK.	12 months	Little's irregularity index (LII), intercanine width.
Gill et al. (2007)	Vacum-Former Retainer	Vacum-Former Retainer	Full-Time = 28 Part-Time = 29	F = 16 M = 12 F = 16 M = 13	FT = 13,7 (2,5) PT = 13,3 (1,4)	No Extraction: 35 Extraction: 65%	Hospital department, London, UK.	6 months	Little's irregularity index (LII), intercanine width.
Kumar et al. (2011)	Vacum-Formed Retainer Begg Retainer	Vacum-Formed Retainer Begg Retainer	VFR = 112 BR = 112	//	//	//	College of Dental Sciences, Davangere, India.	6 months	Little's irregularity index (LII).
O'Rourke et al. (2016)	//	Vacum-Former Retainer Fixed Retainer	VFR = 21 FR = 27	F = 59 M = 23	//	No Extraction: 53,6% Extraction: 46,4%	Hospital, London, UK.	18 months	Little's irregularity index (LII), intercanine width.
Rowland et al. (2006)	Vacum-Former Retainer Hawley Retainer	Vacum-Former Retainer Hawley Retainer	VFR = 201 HR = 196	F = 118 M = 83 F = 123 M = 73	VFR = 14 HR = 15	No Extraction: 66,2% Extraction: 33,8%	Taunton, Bristol, London and Nottingham, UK.	6 months	Little's irregularity index (LII), intercanine width.
Salehi et al. (2013)	Fixed Retainer (PWR) Fixed Retainer (Multi-Stranded)	Fixed Retainer (PWR) Fixed Retainer (Multi-Stranded)	PWR = 68 Multi-stranded = 74	F = 39 M = 29 F = 44 M = 30	PWR = 18.1 (5,2) PT = 18,2 (4,8)	//	School of Dentistry, Shiraz University of Medical Sciences, Iran	18 months	Failure rate.
Shawesh et al. (2009)	Hawley Retainer	Hawley Retainer	Full-Time = 28 Part-Time = 24	F = 58,8% M = 41,2% F = 75,8% M = 24,2%	FT = 15,6 (1,6) PT = 15,8 (1,2)	No Extraction: 17,9% Extraction: 82,1%	Heaton Mersey, Manchester, UK.	12 months	Little's irregularity index (LII).
Störman et al. (2002)	//	Fixed Retainer (0.0195 Respond®) Fixed Retainer (0.0215 Respond®) Fixed Retainer (Prefabricated 3 to 3)	0.0195 Respond®= 31 0.0215 Respond®= 38 Prefabricated 3 to 3 = 34	//	13 to 17	//	Department of Orthodontics, University of Münster, Germany	24 months	Failure rate.

3.3. Risk of Bias Assessment

Although we took only single arm data from the selected studies to perform the meta-analysis, all the pooled data come from RCTs. Therefore, in order to assess the risk of bias, we had to assess the methodological quality of the RCTs; we used the Cochrane Collaboration tool, which is considered the gold standard for this purpose (Table S1). Among the eight studies included for the quantitative synthesis and meta-analysis, only 1 RCT was evaluated to have a high risk of bias [34]. In two RCTs, the risk of bias was unclear [31,33], and five RCTs had a low risk of bias [26–30,32] (Table 3). Consequently, the summary assessments of risk of bias across the studies were considered to be low. The inter-reviewer agreements for risk of bias assessment were suitable, with kappa values of 0.925. Publication bias was not assessed as there were inadequate numbers of included trials to properly develop a funnel plot or more advanced regression-based assessments.

Table 3. Risk of bias assessment.

STUDIES	Risk of Bias						
	Sequence Generation	Allocation Concealment	Blinding of Participants, Personnel and Outcomes	Incomplete Outcome Data	Selective Outcome Reporting	Other Risk of Bias	Overall Risk of Bias
Bolla et al. (2012)	Unclear	Unclear	Unclear	High Risk	Unclear	High Risk	High Risk
Edman et al. (2013)	Low Risk	Low Risk	Low Risk	Low Risk	Low Risk	Low Risk	Low Risk
Egli et al. (2017)	Low Risk	Low Risk	Low Risk	Low Risk	Low Risk	Low Risk	Low Risk
Forde et al. (2017)	Low Risk	Low Risk	Low Risk	Low Risk	Low Risk	Low Risk	Low Risk
Gill et al. (2007)	Low Risk	Low Risk	Low Risk	Low Risk	Low Risk	Low Risk	Low Risk
Kumar et al. (2011)	Unclear	Unclear	Low Risk	Low Risk	Unclear	Unclear	Unclear
O'Rourke et al. (2016)	Low Risk	Low Risk	Low Risk	Low Risk	Low Risk	Low Risk	Low Risk
Rowland et al. (2006)	Low Risk	Low Risk	Low Risk	Low Risk	Unclear	Low Risk	Unclear
Salehi et al. (2013)	Low Risk	Unclear	Low Risk	Low Risk	Low Risk	Low Risk	Unclear
Shawesh et al. (2009)	Low Risk	Low Risk	Low Risk	Low Risk	Low Risk	High Risk	High Risk
Störmann et al. (2002)	Unclear	Unclear	Low Risk	Low Risk	Low Risk	Unclear	Unclear

3.4. Quantitative Data Synthesis

The data showed that the mean difference of intercanine width during the retention period was 0.05 mm (95% CI, −0.41 to 0.51; $P = 0.84$; $I^2 = 99\%$) for the mandibular fixed retainers (Figure 2a), 0.01 mm (95% CI, −0.26 to 0.28; $P = 0.95$; $I^2 = 100\%$) for the mandibular removable retainers (Figure 2b), and −0.13 mm (95% CI, −0.52 to 0.27; $P = 0.53$; $I^2 = 99\%$) for the maxillary removable retainers (Figure 2c). The mean difference of Little's Index during the retention period was 0.48 mm (95% CI, −0.04 to 1.01; $P = 0.07$; $I^2 = 98\%$) for the mandibular fixed retainers (Figure 2d), 0.73 mm (95% CI, 0.47 to 0.98; $P = 0.00001$; $I^2 = 100\%$) for the mandibular removable retainers (Figure 2e), and 0.48 mm (95% CI, 0.27 to 0.68; $P = 0.00001$; $I^2 = 91\%$) for the maxillary removable retainers (Figure 2f).

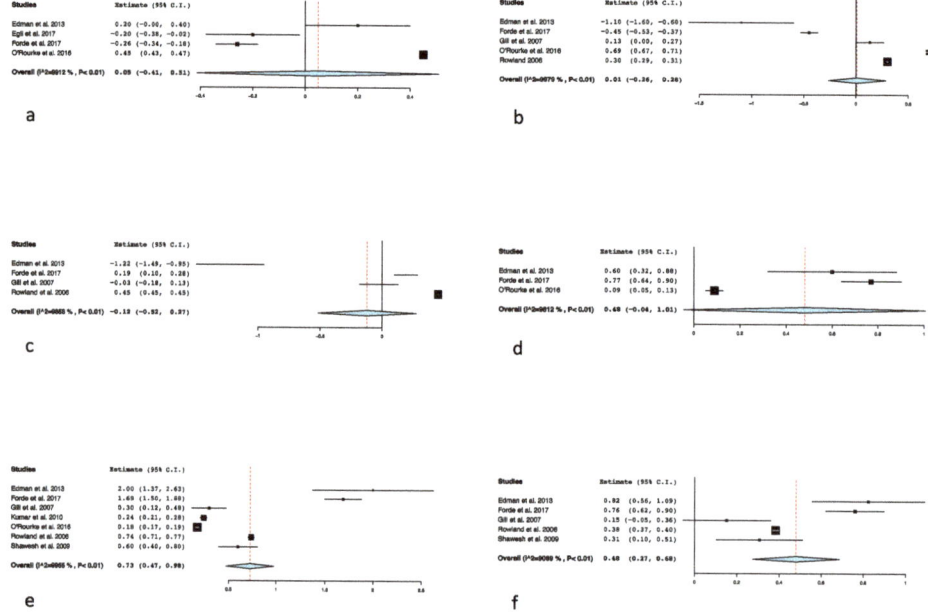

Figure 2. (a) Forest plot of the intercanine width modification: mandibular fixed retainers; (b) mandibular removable retainers; (c) maxillary removable retainers; (d) forest plot of the Little's Index modification: mandibular fixed retainers; (e) mandibular removable retainers; (f) maxillary removable retainers.

3.5. Fixed Retainer Failure Rate

Among the 11 studies included for qualitative synthesis, four RCTs [28,35–37] reported the failure rate of the fixed retainers during the observation period. The summarized failure rate was 41.3% (72/174) for the maxillary arch and 36.7% (115/313) for the mandibular arch (Table 4). Among the four studies, only one RCT had a high risk of bias [35]. For two RCTs, the risk of bias was unclear [36,37], and one RCT had a low risk of bias [28] (Table 3).

Table 4. Fixed retainer failure rate.

	Retainer Characteristics	Maxillary Arch	Mandibular Arch
Bolla et al. (2012)	Glass-Fiber reinforced	4/14 (28.5%)	7/34 (20.5%)
	Multistranded	7/18 (38.8%)	10/32 (31.2%)
Egli et al. (2017)	Direct Bonding	//	11/30 (37%)
	Indirect Bonding	//	13/30 (43%)
Salehi et al. (2013)	Polyethylene Woven Ribbon	27/74 (36.5%)	14/37 (37.8%)
	0.0175 in flexible spiral wire	34/68 (50%)	29/68 (42.6%)
	0.0195 Respond®	//	10/30 (33.3%)
Störmann et al. (2002)	0.0215 Respond®	//	18/36 (50%)
	Prefabricated 3 to 3	//	3/16 (18.7%)
Total		72/174 (41.3%)	115/313 (36.7%)

3.6. Assessment of Quality of Evidence

According to the GRADE [25], there was low level of evidence for all the LII outcomes (Table 5) and for the mandibular and maxillary intercanine width outcomes with both fixed and removable retainers (Table 6). According to the SORT approach [26], the strength of the recommendations was classified as A for LII and C for intercanine width (Table 7).

Table 5. Should fixed retainers or removable retainers be used for maintaining the alignment of anterior teeth?

№ of Studies	Study Design	Certainty Assessment					№ of Patients		Effect		Certainty	Importance
		Risk of Bias	Inconsistency	Indirectness	Imprecision	Other Considerations	Fixed Retainers	Removable Retainers	Relative (95% CI)	Absolute (95% CI)		
Mandibular Fixed												
3	randomised trials	not serious	very serious [a]	not serious	not serious	none	96	96	-	MD 0.48 higher (0.04 lower to 1 higher)	⊕⊕○○ LOW	CRITICAL
Mandibular Removable												
7	randomised trials	very serious [b]	very serious [a]	not serious	not serious	none	818	818	-	MD 0.72 higher (0.47 higher to 0.98 higher)	⊕○○○ VERY LOW	CRITICAL
Maxillary Removable												
5	randomised trials	very serious [c]	very serious [a]	not serious	not serious	none	605	605	-	MD 0.8 higher (0.35 higher to 1.24 higher)	⊕○○○ VERY LOW	CRITICAL
Acrylic Removable Retainers (mandibular)												
3	randomised trials	very serious [b]	very serious [a]	not serious	not serious	none	360	360	-	MD 1.08 higher (0.53 higher to 1.63 higher)	⊕○○○ VERY LOW	CRITICAL
Vacuum-Formed Removable Retainers (mandibular)												
5	randomised trials	serious [d]	very serious [a]	not serious	not serious	none	436	436	-	MD 0.51 higher (0.33 higher to 0.69 higher)	⊕○○○ VERY LOW	CRITICAL

CI: Confidence interval; MD: Mean difference. (**a**) Heterogeneity > 75%; (**b**) in one study, the risk of bias was unclear for "Sequence generation", "Allocation concealment", "Selective Outcome Reporting", and "Other Risk of bias". In one study, the risk of bias was unclear for "Selective Outcome Reporting". In one study, the risk of bias was high for "Other Risk of bias"; (**c**) in one study the risk of bias was unclear for "Selective Outcome Reporting". In one study, the risk of bias was high for "Other Risk of bias"; (**d**) in one study, the risk of bias was unclear for "Sequence generation", "Allocation concealment", "Selective Outcome Reporting", and "Other Risk of bias". In one study, the risk of bias was unclear for "Selective Outcome Reporting".

Table 6. Should fixed retainers or removable retainers be used for maintaining intercanine width?

№ of Studies	Certainty Assessment						№ of Patients		Effect		Certainty	Importance
	Study Design	Risk of Bias	Inconsistency	Indirectness	Imprecision	Other Considerations	Fixed Retainers	Removable Retainers	Relative (95% CI)	Absolute (95% CI)		
Mandibular Fixed												
4	randomised trials	not serious	very serious [a]	not serious	not serious	none	126	126	-	MD 0.05 higher (0.41 lower to 0.51 higher)	⊕⊕○○ LOW	CRITICAL
Mandibular Removable												
5	randomised trials	not serious	very serious [a]	not serious	not serious	none	542	542	-	MD 0.01 higher (0.27 lower to 0.28 higher)	⊕⊕○○ LOW	CRITICAL
Maxillary Removable												
4	randomised trials	not serious	very serious [a]	not serious	not serious	none	553	553	-	MD 0.13 lower (0.52 lower to 0.27 higher)	⊕⊕○○ LOW	CRITICAL

CI: Confidence interval; MD: Mean difference. (a) Heterogeneity > 75%.

Table 7. Strength of recommendations for each outcome investigated in the present study.

Outcomes	Study Quality *	Consistency *	Strength of Recommendation *	Explanation
Intercanine width				
Mandibular fixed retainer	Level 3	Yes	C	Disease-oriented outcome Meta-analysis including 4 RCTs
Mandibular removable retainer	Level 3	Yes	C	Disease-oriented outcome Meta-analysis including 5 RCTs
Maxillary removable retainer	Level 3	Yes	C	Disease-oriented outcome Meta-analysis including 4 RCTs
Irregularity Index				
Mandibular fixed retainer	Level 1	Yes	A	Patient-oriented outcome Meta-analysis including 3 RCTs
Mandibular removable retainer	Level 1	Yes	A	Patient-oriented outcome Meta-analysis including 7 RCTs
Maxillary removable retainer	Level 1	Yes	A	Patient-oriented outcome Meta-analysis including 5 RCTs
Acrylic removable retainer	Level 1	Yes	A	Disease-oriented outcome Meta-analysis including 3 RCTs
Vacuum-Formed Removable retainer	Level 1	Yes	A	Disease-oriented outcome Meta-analysis including 5 RCTs

* Reports of the levels of study quality, consistency of measured outcomes, and strength of recommendations according to the Strength of Recommendation Taxonomy (SORT) system.

4. Discussion

To the best of our knowledge, this is the first review with meta-analysis that investigates the current literature with the best evidence (RCTs) on the efficacy of orthodontic retainers to maintain the occlusal results after fixed orthodontic treatment. The results of this meta-analysis will provide clinicians a quantitative evaluation of the efficacy of fixed and removable retainers and consequently a quantitative evaluation of orthodontic relapse during the retention period.

The pooled data show that the intercanine width does not change significantly during retention with all evaluated retention appliances [37–44].

The data show that the fixed retainers are also able to avoid significant modifications of LII ($p = 0.07$). However, this datum should be interpreted with caution because of the fewer number of considered trials. Conversely, the use of removable retainers showed a significant increase of LII. This datum was obtained by pooling the data from five trials for the maxillary arch (Figure 2f) and from seven trials for the mandibular arch (Figure 2e); it can be considered a consistent meta-analytic datum. The amount of variation for LII is 0.48 and 0.72 mm, respectively, for the maxillary and mandibular arch. This result clearly shows that, despite the use of a removable retainer appliance, the teeth of both arches present a small statistically significant (but clinically insignificant) alignment alteration. These results, especially for intercanine width, must be interpreted with caution due to the young age of the sample participants, as this type of alteration can influence the outcome due to residual growth and patient compliance.

Interestingly, our data show a significant alteration of LII in the absence of modification of the intercanine width. These results could be explained by interpreting the alteration of LII as a consequence of a single tooth rotational relapse, rather than a transversal inter-canine diameter relapse. The reported modifications of LII could be related to specific factors associated with the use of removable retainers, such as patient compliance and the limitations of using retainers nocturnally. This last hypothesis, however, does not seem to be supported by the evidence. Indeed, one of the considered RCTs compared removable retainers used full time and removable retainers used part-time [45–55]. The authors did not find significant differences in terms of relapse after 12 months of retention.

Compliance is certainly an issue related to removable retainers. However, the results of this review clearly show that fixed retainers are not free of issues. In fact, the failure rate of fixed retainers (caused by wire breakage or bonding failure) is, on average, 41% and 36% for maxillary and mandibular retainers, respectively (Table 4). These data are in accordance with previously published data [14,56–61].

One limitation of this meta-analysis is the small number of included trials; this aspect affected the I2 index, undervaluing the extent of between-study heterogeneity [62,63]. The I2 values reported a high total variation across the studies, with a mean value and a standard deviation equal to 97.8% and 2.2%, respectively. This variation was assumed to be due to the clinical heterogeneity of the different appliances used in the considered RCTs. Moreover, the source of heterogeneity could be related to other factors such as patient compliance, final occlusal results, orthodontist expertise, type of malocclusion, and type of treatment (with or without extractions) [13,64–77].

The I2 values potentially affected the level of evidence of our findings, which ranged from very low to low, according to the GRADE approach. Although we selected only published trials offering the highest level of evidence (RCTs), the GRADE score showed that the included studies provided, in most cases, a very low quality of evidence (Tables 5 and 6). This result should be assessed while considering the difficulties in conducting RCTs for orthodontics [46].

All these aspects increased the heterogeneity of the different clinical trials and, consequently, contributed to limiting the methodological GRADE score of the orthodontic trials.

The SORT approach (Table 7) revealed a high strength of recommendations for the LII outcome and a poor strength of recommendations for the intercanine width outcome, likely because the LII represents a clinical outcome that directly affect smile aesthetics and appearance (i.e., a patient-oriented outcome).

The sensitivity analysis showed a similar outcome compared with the results of this meta-analysis for the same parameter (0.74) (95% Cl, 0.47 to 1.01; $P = 0.00001$; $I^2 = 100\%$), confirming the validity of the performed meta-analysis.

5. Conclusions

The results of this meta-analysis show that all the considered retainers are effective in maintaining dental alignment after fixed orthodontic treatment. However, the fixed retainers showed greater efficacy than the removable retainers.

The most important issues for fixed and removable retainers are, respectively, the risk of failure and patient compliance. Further RCT studies with longer observation periods are needed in order to assess the long-term efficacy of orthodontic retainers.

Supplementary Materials: The following are available online at http://www.mdpi.com/2076-3417/10/9/3107/s1, Table S1: Excluded articles with reason for exclusion. Figure S1: Sensitivity analysis.

Author Contributions: Conceptualization, A.L.G. and L.R.; methodology, M.P., G.I.; software, V.R.; writing—original draft preparation, writing—review and editing R.N. and G.I. All authors have read and agreed to the published version of the manuscript.

Funding: This research received no external funding.

Conflicts of Interest: The authors declare no conflict of interest.

References

1. Little, R.M.; Wallen, T.R.; Riedel, R.A. Stability and relapse of mandibular anterior alignment—First premolar extraction cases treated by traditional edgewise orthodontics. *Am. J. Orthod.* **1981**, *80*, 349–365. [CrossRef]
2. Blake, M.; Bibby, K. Retention and stability: A review of the literature. *Am. J. Orthod. Dentofac. Orthop.* **1998**, *114*, 299–306. [CrossRef]
3. Nucera, R.; Lo Giudice, A.; Bellocchio, M.; Spinuzza, P.; Caprioglio, A.; Cordasco, G. Diagnostic concordance between skeletal cephalometrics, radiographbased soft-tissue cephalometrics, and photograph-based soft-tissue cephalometrics. *Eur. J. Orthod.* **2017**, *39*, 352–357. [PubMed]

4. Lo Giudice, A.; Nucera, R.; Leonardi, R.; Paiusco, A.; Baldoni, M.; Caccianiga, G. A Comparative Assessment of the Efficiency of Orthodontic Treatment with and without Photobiomodulation during Mandibular Decrowding in Young Subjects: A Single-Center, Single-Blind Randomized Controlled Trial. *Photobiomodul Photomed. Laser Surg.* **2020**. [CrossRef] [PubMed]
5. Richardson, M.E. Late lower arch crowding in relation to primary crowding. *Angle Orthod.* **1982**, *44*, 56–61.
6. Lo Giudice, A.; Nucera, R.; Perillo, L.; Paiusco, A.; Caccianiga, G. Is low-level laser therapy an effective method to alleviate pain induced by active orthodontic alignment archwire? A randomized clinical trial. *J. Evid. Based Dent. Prac.* **2019**, *19*, 71–78. [CrossRef]
7. Richardson, M.E. Late lower arch crowding in relation to the direction of eruption. *Eur. J. Orthod.* **1996**, *18*, 341–347. [CrossRef]
8. Bondemark, L.; Holm, A.K.; Hansen, K.; Axelsson, S.; Mohlin, B.; Brattstrom, V.; Paulin, G.; Pietila, T. Long term stability of orthodontic treatment and patient satisfaction: A systematic review. *Angle Orthod.* **2007**, *77*, 181–191. [CrossRef]
9. Weiland, F. The role of occlusal discrepancies in the long-term stability of the mandibular arch. *Eur. J. Orthod.* **1994**, *16*, 521–529. [CrossRef]
10. Little, R.M.; Riedel, R.A. Postretention evaluation of stability and relapse—Mandibular arches with generalized spacing. *Am. J. Orthod. Dentofac. Orthop.* **1989**, *95*, 37–41. [CrossRef]
11. Littlewood, S.J.; Millett, D.T.; Doubleday, B.; Bearn, D.R.; Worthington, H.V. Retention procedures for stabilising tooth position after treatment with orthodontic braces. *Cochrane Database Syst. Rev.* **2016**. [CrossRef]
12. Al-Moghrabi, D.; Pandis, N.; Fleming, P.S. The effects of fixed and removable orthodontic retainers: A systematic review. *Prog. Orthod.* **2016**, *17*, 24. [CrossRef] [PubMed]
13. Nucera, R.; Gatto, E.; Borsellino, C.; Aceto, P.; Fabiano, F.; Matarese, G.; Perillo, L.; Cordasco, G. Influence of bracket-slot design on the forces released by superelastic nickel-titanium alignment wires in different deflection configurations. *Angle Orthod.* **2014**, *84*, 541–547. [CrossRef] [PubMed]
14. Lo Giudice, G.; Lo Giudice, A.; Isola, G.; Fabiano, F.; Artemisia, A.; Fabiano, V.; Nucera, R.; Matarese, G. Evaluation of bond strength and detachment interface distribution of different bracket base designs. *Acta Med. Mediterr.* **2015**, *31*, 585–590.
15. Papadopoulos, M.A. Meta-analysis in evidence-based orthodontics. *Orthod. Craniofac. Res* **2003**, *6*, 112–126. [CrossRef]
16. Nucera, R.; Militi, A.; Lo Giudice, A.; Longo, V.; Fastuca, R.; Caprioglio, A.; Cordasco, G.; Papadopoulos, M.A. Skeletal and Dental Effectiveness of Treatment of Class II Malocclusion with Headgear: A Systematic Review and Meta-analysis. *J. Evid. Based Dent. Prac.* **2018**, *18*, 41–58. [CrossRef]
17. Higgins, J.P.T.; Green, S. (Eds.) *Cochrane Handbook for Systematic Reviews of Interventions*, (version 5.1.0, updated March 2016); The Cochrane Collaboration: London, UK, 2016.
18. Nucera, R.; Lo Giudice, A.; Rustico, L.; Matarese, G.; Papadopoulos, M.A.; Cordasco, G. Effectiveness of orthodontic treatment with functional appliances on maxillary growth in the short term: A systematic review and meta-analysis. *Am. J. Orthod. Dentofac. Orthop.* **2016**, *149*, 600–611.e3. [CrossRef]
19. Liberati, A.; Altman, D.G.; Tetzlaff, J.; Mulrow, C.; Gotzsche, P.C.; Ioannidis, J.P.A.; Clarke, M.; Devereaux, P.J.; Kleijnen, J.; Moher, D. The PRISMA statement for reporting systematic reviews and meta-analyses of studies that evaluate health care interventions: Explanation and elaboration. *J. Clin. Epidemiol.* **2009**, *62*, e1–e34. [CrossRef]
20. Fitzpatrick-Lewis, D.; Ciliska, D.; Thomas, H. *The Methods for the Synthesis of Studies without Control Groups*; National Collaborating Centre for Methods and Tools: Hamilton, ON, Canada, 2009.
21. Chambers, D.; Rodgers, M.; Woolacott, N. Not only randomized controlled trials, but also case series should be considered in systematic reviews of rapidly developing technologies. *J. Clin. Epidemiol.* **2009**, *62*, 1253–1260.e4. [CrossRef]
22. Dalziel, K.; Round, A.; Stein, K.; Garside, R.; Castelnuovo, E.; Payne, L. Do the findings of case series studies vary significantly according to methodological characteristics? *Health Technol Assess.* **2005**, *9*, 1–148. [CrossRef]
23. Hozo, S.L.; Djulbegovic, B.; Hozo, I. Estimating the mean and variance from the median, range, and the size of a sample. *BMC Med. Res. Methodol.* **2005**, *5*, 13. [CrossRef] [PubMed]

24. Wallace, B.C.; Dahabreh, I.J.; Trikalinos, T.A.; Lau, J.; Trow, P.; Schmid, C.H. Closing the Gap between Methodologists and End-Users: R as a Computational Back-End. *J. Stat. Softw.* **2012**, *49*, 1–15. [CrossRef]
25. Falck-Ytter, Y.; Guyatt, G.H.; Vist, G.; Kunz, R. Rating quality of evidence and strength of recommendations GRADE: An emerging consensus on rating quality of evidence and strength of recommendations. *BMJ* **2008**, *336*, 924–926.
26. Newman, M.G.; Weyant, R.; Hujoel, P. JEBDP improves grading system and adopts strength of recommendation taxonomy grading (SORT) for guidelines and systematic reviews. *J. Evid. Based Dent. Prac.* **2007**, *7*, 147–150. [CrossRef] [PubMed]
27. Edman Tynelius, G.; Bondemark, L.; Lilja-Karlander, E. A randomized controlled trial of three orthodontic retention methods in Class I four premolar extraction cases—Stability after 2 years in retention. *Orthod. Craniofac. Res.* **2013**, *16*, 105–115. [CrossRef] [PubMed]
28. Egli, F.; Bovali, E.; Kiliaridis, S.; Cornelis, M.A. Indirect vs direct bonding of mandibular fixed retainers in orthodontic patients: Comparison of retainer failures and posttreatment stability. A 2-year follow-up of a single-center randomized controlled trial. *Am. J. Orthod. Dentofac. Orthop.* **2017**, *151*, 15–27. [CrossRef]
29. Forde, K.; Storey, M.; Littlewood, S.J.; Paul Scott, P.; Luther, F.; Kang, J. Bonded versus vacuum-formed retainers: A randomized controlled trial. Part 1: Stability, retainer survival, and patient satisfaction outcomes after 12 months. *Eur. J. Orthod.* **2018**, *40*, 387–398. [CrossRef]
30. Gill, D.S.; Naini, F.B.; Jones, A.; Tredwin, C.J. Part-time versus full-time retainer wear following fixed appliance therapy: A randomized prospective controlled trial. *World J. Orthod.* **2007**, *8*, 300–306.
31. Kumar, A.G.; Bansal, A. Effectiveness and acceptability of Essix and Begg retainers: A prospective study. *Aust. Orthod. J.* **2011**, *27*, 52–56.
32. O'Rourke, N.; Albeedh, H.; Sharma, P.; Johal, A. Effectiveness of bonded and vacuum-formed retainers: A prospective randomized controlled clinical trial. *Am. J. Orthod. Dentofac. Orthop.* **2016**, *150*, 406–415. [CrossRef]
33. Rowland, H.; Hichens, L.; Williams, A.; Hills, D.; Killingback, N. The effectiveness of Hawley and vacuum-formed retainers: A single-center randomized controlled trial. *Am. J. Orthod. Dentofac. Orthop.* **2007**, *132*, 730–737. [CrossRef]
34. Shawesh, M.; Bhatti, B.; Usmani, T.; Mandall, N. Hawley retainers full- or part-time? A randomized clinical trial. *Eur. J. Orthod.* **2010**, *32*, 165–170. [CrossRef]
35. Bolla, E.; Cozzani, M.; Doldo, T.; Fontana, M. Failure evaluation after a 6-year retention period: A comparison between glass fiber-reinforced (GFR) and multistranded bonded retainers. *Int. Orthod.* **2012**, *10*, 16–28. [CrossRef] [PubMed]
36. Salehi, P.; Zarif Najafi, H.; Roeinpeikar, S.M. Comparison of survival time between two types of orthodontic fixed retainer: A prospective randomized clinical trial. *Prog. Orthod.* **2013**, *14*, 25. [CrossRef] [PubMed]
37. Störmann, I.; Ehmer, U. A prospective randomized study of different retainer types. *J. Orofac. Orthop.* **2002**, *63*, 42–50. [CrossRef] [PubMed]
38. Isola, G.; Anastasi, G.P.; Matarese, G.; Williams, R.C.; Cutroneo, G.; Bracco, P.; Piancino, M.G. Functional and molecular outcomes of the human masticatory muscles. *Oral Dis.* **2018**, *24*, 1428–1441. [CrossRef]
39. Isola, G.; Polizzi, A.; Santonocito, S.; Alibrandi, A.; Ferlito, S. Expression of Salivary and Serum Malondialdehyde and Lipid Profile of Patients with Periodontitis and Coronary Heart Disease. *Int. J. Mol. Sci.* **2019**, *20*, 6061. [CrossRef]
40. Isola, G.; Perillo, L.; Migliorati, M.; Matarese, M.; Dalessandri, D.; Grassia, V.; Alibrandi, A.; Matarese, G. The impact of temporomandibular joint arthritis on functional disability and global health in patients with juvenile idiopathic arthritis. *Eur. J. Orthod.* **2019**, *41*, 117–124. [CrossRef]
41. Mev, J. Are random controlled trials appropriate for orthodontics? *Evid. Based Dent.* **2002**, *3*, 35–36.
42. Leonardi, R.; Lo Giudice, A.; Rugeri, M.; Muraglie, S.; Cordasco, G.; Barbato, E. Three-dimensional evaluation on digital casts of maxillary palatal size and morphology in patients with functional posterior crossbite. *Eur. J. Orthod.* **2018**, *40*, 556–562. [CrossRef]
43. Leonardi, R. Cone-beam computed tomography and three-dimensional orthodontics. Where we are and future perspectives. *J. Orthod.* **2019**, *46* (Suppl. 1), 45–48. [CrossRef] [PubMed]
44. Caccianiga, G.; Crestale, C.; Cozzani, M.; Piras, A.; Mutinelli, S.; Lo Giudice, A.; Cordasco, G. Low-level laser therapy and invisible removal aligners. *J. Biol. Regul. Homeost. Agents* **2016**, *30* (Suppl. 1), 107–113. [PubMed]

45. Isola, G.; Alibrandi, A.; Rapisarda, E.; Matarese, G.; Williams, R.C.; Leonardi, R. Association of vitamin d in patients with periodontal and cardiovascular disease: A cross-sectional study. *J. Periodontal. Res.* **2020**. [CrossRef]
46. Isola, G.; Alibrandi, A.; Currò, M.; Matarese, M.; Ricca, S.; Matarese, G.; Ientile, R.; Kocher, T. Evaluation of salivary and serum ADMA levels in patients with periodontal and cardiovascular disease as subclinical marker of cardiovascular risk. *J. Periodontol.* **2020**. [CrossRef]
47. Isola, G.; Polizzi, A.; Alibrandi, A.; Indelicato, F.; Ferlito, S. Analysis of Endothelin-1 concentrations in individuals with periodontitis. *Sci. Rep.* **2020**. [CrossRef] [PubMed]
48. Isola, G.; Matarese, G.; Ramaglia, L.; Pedullà, E.; Rapisarda, E.; Iorio-Siciliano, V. Association between periodontitis and glycosylated haemoglobin before diabetes onset: A cross-sectional study. *Clin. Oral Investig.* 2019. [CrossRef]
49. Cutroneo, G.; Piancino, M.G.; Ramieri, G.; Bracco, P.; Vita, G.; Isola, G.; Vermiglio, G.; Favaloro, A.; Anastasi, G.; Trimarchi, F. Expression of muscle-specific integrins in masseter muscle fibers during malocclusion disease. *Int. J. Mol. Med.* **2012**, *30*, 235–242. [CrossRef]
50. Isola, G.; Matarese, M.; Ramaglia, L.; Cicciù, M.; Matarese, G. Evaluation of the efficacy of celecoxib and ibuprofen on postoperative pain, swelling, and mouth opening after surgical removal of impacted third molars: A randomized, controlled clinical trial. *Int. J. Oral Maxillofac. Surg.* **2019**, *48*, 1348–1354. [CrossRef]
51. Isola, G.; Alibrandi, A.; Pedullà, E.; Grassia, V.; Ferlito, S.; Perillo, L.; Rapisarda, E. Analysis of the Effectiveness of Lornoxicam and Flurbiprofen on Management of Pain and Sequelae Following Third Molar Surgery: A Randomized, Controlled, Clinical Trial. *J. Clin. Med.* **2019**, *8*, 325. [CrossRef]
52. Isola, G.; Matarese, G.; Alibrandi, A.; Dalessandri, D.; Migliorati, M.; Pedullà, E.; Rapisarda, E. Comparison of Effectiveness of Etoricoxib and Diclofenac on Pain and Perioperative Sequelae After Surgical Avulsion of Mandibular Third Molars: A Randomized, Controlled, Clinical Trial. *Clin. J. Pain* **2019**, *35*, 908–915. [CrossRef]
53. Lo Giudice, A.; Brewer, I.; Leonardi, R.; Roberts, N.; Bagnato, G.5. Pain threshold and temporomandibular function in systemic sclerosis: Comparison with psoriatic arthritis. *Clin. Rheumatol.* **2018**, *37*, 1861–1867. [CrossRef] [PubMed]
54. Lo Giudice, A.; Nucera, R.; Matarese, G.; Portelli, M.; Cervino, G.; Lo Giudice, G.; Militi, A.; Caccianiga, G.; Cicciù, M.; Cordasco, G. Analysis of resistance to sliding expressed during first order correction with conventional and self-ligating brackets: An in-vitro study. *Int. J. Clin. Exp. Med.* **2016**, *9*, 15575–15581.
55. Piancino, M.G.; Isola, G.; Cannavale, R.; Cutroneo, G.; Vermiglio, G.; Bracco, P.; Anastasi, G.P. From periodontal mechanoreceptors to chewing motor control: A systematic review. *Arch. Oral Biol.* **2017**, *78*, 109–121. [CrossRef] [PubMed]
56. Perillo, L.; Padricelli, G.; Isola, G.; Femiano, F.; Chiodini, P.; Matarese, G. Class II malocclusion division 1:.A new classification method by cephalometric analysis. *Eur. J. Paediatr. Dent.* **2012**, *13*, 192–196.
57. Isola, G.; Giudice, A.L.; Polizzi, A.; Alibrandi, A.; Patini, R.; Ferlito, S. Periodontitis and Tooth Loss Have Negative Systemic Impact on Circulating Progenitor Cell Levels: A Clinical Study. *Genes* **2019**, *10*, 1022. [CrossRef]
58. Isola, G.; Polizzi, A.; Muraglie, S.; Leonardi, R.M.; Lo Giudice, A. Assessment Of vitamin C And Antioxidants Profiles In Saliva And Serum In Patients With Periodontitis And Ischemic Heart Disease. *Nutrients* **2019**, *11*, 2956. [CrossRef]
59. Cannavale, R.; Matarese, G.; Isola, G.; Grassia, V.; Perillo, L. Early treatment of an ectopic premolar to prevent molar-premolar transposition. *Am. J. Orthod. Dentofac. Orthop.* **2013**, *143*, 559–569. [CrossRef]
60. Lo Giudice, A.; Barbato, E.; Cosentino, L.; Ferraro, C.M.; Leonardi, R. Alveolar bone changes after rapid maxillary expansion with tooth-born appliances: A systematic review. *Eur J Orthod.* **2018**, *40*, 296–303. [CrossRef]
61. Isola, G.; Matarese, M.; Briguglio, F.; Grassia, V.; Picciolo, G.; Fiorillo, L.; Matarese, G. Effectiveness of Low-Level Laser Therapy during Tooth Movement: A Randomized Clinical Trial. *Materials* **2019**, *12*, 2187. [CrossRef]
62. Lo Giudice, A.; Rustico, L.; Caprioglio, A.; Migliorati, M.; Nucera, R. Evaluation of condylar cortical bone thickness in patient groups with different vertical facial dimensions using cone-beam computed tomography. *Odontology* **2020**, in press. [CrossRef]

63. Lo Giudice, A.; Fastuca, R.; Portelli, M.; Militi, A.; Bellocchio, M.; Spinuzza, P.; Briguglio, F.; Caprioglio, A.; Nucera, R. Effects of rapid vs slow maxillary expansion on nasal cavity dimensions in growing subjects: A methodological and reproducibility study. *Eur. J. Paediatr. Dent.* **2017**, *18*, 299–304. [PubMed]
64. Caccianiga, G.; Paiusco, A.; Perillo, L.; Nucera, R.; Pinsino, A.; Maddalone, M.; Cordasco, G.; Lo Giudice, A. Does Low-Level Laser Therapy Enhance the Efficiency of Orthodontic Dental Alignment? Results from a Randomized Pilot Study. *Photomed Laser Surg.* **2017**, *35*, 421–426. [CrossRef] [PubMed]
65. Matarese, G.; Portelli, M.; Mazza, M.; Militi, A.; Nucera, R.; Gatto, E.; Cordasco, G. Evaluation of skin dose in a low dose spiral CT protocol. *Eur. J. Paediatr. Dent.* **2006**, *7*, 77–80.
66. Caprioglio, A.; Bergamini, C.; Franchi, L.; Vercellini, N.; Zecca, P.A. ; Nucera R, Fastuca R Prediction of Class II improvement after rapid maxillary expansion in early mixed dentition. *Prog. Orthod.* **2017**, *18*, 9. [CrossRef] [PubMed]
67. Nucera, R.; Lo Giudice, A.; Matarese, G.; Artemisia, A.; Cordasco, G.; Bramanti, E. Analysis of the characteristics of slot design affecting resistance to sliding during active archwire configurations. *Prog Orthod.* **2013**, *14*, 35. [CrossRef] [PubMed]
68. Isola, G.; Matarese, G.; Cordasco, G.; Rotondo, F.; Crupi, A.; Ramaglia, L. Anticoagulant therapy in patients undergoing dental interventions: A critical review of the literature and current perspectives. *Minerva Stomatol.* **2015**, *64*, 21–46.
69. Matarese, G.; Isola, G.; Anastasi, G.P.; Cutroneo, G.; Favaloro, A.; Vita, G.; Cordasco, G.; Milardi, D.; Zizzari, V.L.; Tetè, S.; et al. Transforming Growth Factor Beta 1 and Vascular Endothelial Growth Factor levels in the pathogenesis of periodontal disease. *Eur. J. Inflamm.* **2013**, *11*, 479–488. [CrossRef]
70. Isola, G.; Williams, R.C.; Lo Gullo, A.; Ramaglia, L.; Matarese, M.; Iorio-Siciliano, V.; Cosio, C.; Matarese, G. Risk association between scleroderma disease characteristics, periodontitis, and tooth loss. *Clin. Rheumatol.* **2017**, *36*, 2733–2741. [CrossRef]
71. Matarese, G.; Isola, G.; Alibrandi, A.; Lo Gullo, A.; Bagnato, G.; Cordasco, G.; Perillo, L. Occlusal and MRI characterizations in systemic sclerosis patients: A prospective study from Southern Italian cohort. *Joint. Bone. Spine.* **2016**, *83*, 57–62. [CrossRef]
72. Ametrano, G.; D'Antò, V.; Di Caprio, M.P.; Simeone, M.; Rengo, S.; Spagnuolo, G. Effects of sodium hypochlorite and ethylenediaminetetraacetic acid on rotary nickel-titanium instruments evaluated using atomic force microscopy. *Int. Endod. J.* **2011**, *44*, 203–209. [CrossRef]
73. Spagnuolo, G.; Ametrano, G.; D'Antò, V.; Formisano, A.; Simeone, M.; Riccitiello, F.; Amato, M.; Rengo, S. Microcomputed tomography analysis of mesiobuccal orifices and major apical foramen in first maxillary molars. *Open. Dent. J.* **2012**, *6*, 118–125. [CrossRef] [PubMed]
74. Krifka, S.; Petzel, C.; Bolay, C.; Hiller, K.A.; Spagnuolo, G.; Schmalz, G.; Schweikl, H. Activation of stress-regulated transcription factors by triethylene glycol dimethacrylate monomer. *Biomaterials* **2011**, *32*, 1787–1795. [CrossRef] [PubMed]
75. Pelo, S.; Saponaro, G.; Patini, R.; Staderini, E.; Giordano, A.; Gasparini, G.; Garagiola, U.; Azzuni, C.; Cordaro, M.; Foresta, E.; et al. Risks in surgery-first orthognathic approach: Complications of segmental osteotomies of the jaws. A systematic review. *Eur. Rev. Med. Pharmacol. Sci.* **2017**, *21*, 4–12. [PubMed]
76. Facciolo, M.T.; Riva, F.; Gallenzi, P.; Patini, R.; Gaglioti, D. A rare case of oral multisystem Langerhans cell histiocytosis. *J. Clin. Expd. Dent.* **2017**, *9*, e820–e824. [CrossRef]
77. Cordasco, G.; Lo Giudice, A.; Militi, A.; Nucera, R.; Triolo, G.; Matarese, G. In vitro evaluation of resistance to sliding in self-ligating and conventional bracket systems during dental alignment. *Korean J. Orthod.* **2012**, *42*, 218–224. [CrossRef]

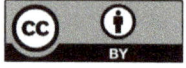

© 2020 by the authors. Licensee MDPI, Basel, Switzerland. This article is an open access article distributed under the terms and conditions of the Creative Commons Attribution (CC BY) license (http://creativecommons.org/licenses/by/4.0/).

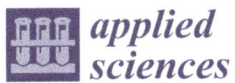

Article

Analysis of Chronic Periodontitis in Tonsillectomy Patients: A Longitudinal Follow-Up Study Using a National Health Screening Cohort

Soo Hwan Byun [1], Chanyang Min [2,3], Yong Bok Kim [4], Heejin Kim [4], Sung Hun Kang [5], Bum Jung Park [6], Ji Hye Wee [6], Hyo Geun Choi [2,6,*] and Seok Jin Hong [4,*]

1. Department of Oral & Maxillofacial Surgery, Dentistry, Sacred Heart Hospital, Hallym University College of Medicine, Anyang 14068, Korea; purheit@daum.net
2. Hallym Data Science Laboratory, Hallym University College of Medicine, 14068 Anyang, Korea; joicemin@naver.com
3. Graduate School of Public Health, Seoul National University, Seoul 03080, Korea
4. Department of Otorhinolaryngology-Head & Neck Surgery, Dongtan Sacred Heart Hospital, Hallym University College of Medicine, Dongtan 18450, Korea; yongbok@hallym.or.kr (Y.B.K.); mir5020@hallym.or.kr (H.K.)
5. Department of Biomedical Sciences, College of Medicine, Hallym University, Chuncheon 24252, Korea; malice23@nate.com
6. Department of Otorhinolaryngology-Head & Neck Surgery, Sacred Heart Hospital, Hallym University College of Medicine, Anyang 14068, Korea; bumjung426@gmail.com (B.J.P.); weejh07@gmail.com (J.H.W.)
* Correspondence: pupen@naver.com (H.G.C.); enthsj@hanmail.net (S.J.H.); Tel.: +82-10-9033-9224 (H.G.C.); +82-31-8086-2670 (S.J.H.)

Received: 31 March 2020; Accepted: 19 May 2020; Published: 25 May 2020

Abstract: This study aimed to compare the risk of chronic periodontitis (CP) between participants who underwent tonsillectomy and those who did not (control participants) using a national cohort dataset. Patients who underwent tonsillectomy were selected from a total of 514,866 participants. A control group was included if participants had not undergone tonsillectomy from 2002 to 2015. The number of CP treatments was counted from the date of the tonsillectomy treatment. Patients who underwent tonsillectomy were matched 1:4 with control participants who were categorized based on age, sex, income, and region of residence. Finally, 1044 patients who underwent tonsillectomy were matched 1:4 with 4176 control participants. The adjusted estimated value of the number of post-index date (ID) CP did not reach statistical significance in any post-ID year (each of $p > 0.05$). In another subgroup analysis according to the number of pre- ID CP, it did not show statistical significance. This study revealed that tonsillectomy was not strongly associated with reducing the risk of CP. Even though the tonsils and periodontium are located adjacently, and tonsillectomy and CP may be related to bacterial inflammation, there was no significant risk of CP in patients undergoing tonsillectomy.

Keywords: tonsillectomy; chronic periodontitis; cohort; Korea

1. Introduction

Periodontitis is inflammation around the teeth and alveolar bone that causes destruction of the surrounding structures [1]. Bacterial microorganisms in the subgingival area are generally thought to be the main etiological factor in the development of periodontitis [2]. Bacterial microorganisms— such as *Tanerella forsythia*, *Treponema denticola*, and *Porphyromonas gingivalis*—are related to chronic periodontitis [3,4]. Socransky et al. reported that bacteria such as *Fusobacterium nucleatum*, *Peptostreptococcus micros*, *Campylobacter rectus*, and *Eubacterium nodatum* could be factors for periodontitis [3]. Periodontal inflammation could be worsened by systemic factors such as general diseases and tobacco use [5–9]. Previous studies have shown that periodontitis can cause reactions in the immune system and a variety of diseases, including IgA nephropathy and glycosylated haemoglobin leading to diabetes onset [10–12]. Isola et al. reported that patients with chronic periodontitis (CP) exhibited significantly lower serum levels of vitamin D compared to the healthy controls [13]. The study showed that low serum vitamin D levels correlated with tooth loss and periodontitis, especially in CP patients. Evaluation of vitamin D levels should be recommended at the beginning of periodontal treatment as it can predict and decrease the risk of CP aggravation [13,14].

Periodontitis is difficult to control and can be managed with periodontal treatment to maintain the present condition and prevent further deterioration. Biofilms should be removed, and oral hygiene training should be conducted to reduce the production of new biofilms [15]. Regeneration for the loss of the alveolar bone and gingiva has been attempted with various types of surgical flaps, bone grafting, guided generation, enamel matrix protein, and laser treatment [16]. However, the attempts have not been satisfactory; therefore, many studies have been conducted from various perspectives attempting to assist with regeneration.

Several studies have been conducted that focus on periodontal treatment, including the use of pharmaceutics, such as the application of topical antiseptics (povidone-iodine or chlorhexidine) [15,17]. Quirynen et al. proposed Full Mouth Disinfection (FMD), a treatment that focuses on the disinfection of all the intraoral niches including the periodontal pockets, dorsum of the tongue, and palatine tonsils [18]. According to the FMD proposal, it is vital to prevent microbial reinfection of the previously treated periodontium and niches. Therefore, meticulous scaling within 24 h was proposed, followed by repeated disinfection of all the intraoral niches [18].

A tonsillectomy is usually performed for the treatment of chronic tonsillitis or sleep apnea [19]. It is also recommended for periodic fever, peritonsillar abscess, guttate psoriasis, aphthous stomatitis, and tonsil cancer. There is sufficient evidence that tonsillectomy does not have a significant negative effect on the immune system [19,20]. The majority of studies have reported that the procedure does not appear to affect the long-term risk of infection [21]. On the contrary, some studies have demonstrated changes in immunoglobulin concentrations following tonsillectomy [19]. Bacterial activity determines the level of inflammation, ulceration, or necrosis of the palatine tonsils. These inflammatory or pathologic disorders related to the tonsils are common causes of tonsillectomy.

The palatine tonsils are located in the oropharynx, close to the intraoral area, and it is assumed that the transmission of bacteria can occur between these areas [22]. The relationship between the anatomic position of the tonsils and the intraoral area is believed to explain why tonsillectomy and periodontitis may exhibit similar bacteriologic and clinical properties. In a previous study, periodontal pathogens were detected in the tonsillar area of periodontitis patients [23]. The palatine tonsils have already been suggested as the source of reinfection for previously treated periodontal areas [17]. Biofilms in the subgingival area and saliva exhibited the highest similarity to that of the tonsils in the study [23]. Anaerobic bacteria of the intraoral area—such as *Porphyromonas gingivalis* and *Fusobacterium nucleatum*—was found to be similar to the bacteria of the oropharyngeal area in previous studies [8]. *Prevotella intermedia* and *Treponema denticola* were also found more frequently in infected subgingival pockets [24,25]. While these bacteria are rarely found in a normal periodontium, they are usually present in periodontitis. Similarly, these anaerobic bacteria were found in tonsils with recurrent inflammation [25]. The present study was designed based on the anatomic nearness and bacterial similarity indicated in previous studies, suggesting the possibility of an association between the palatine tonsil area and periodontitis [18,22,24–26].

Despite the validity of those previous studies, the clinical association between tonsillectomy and periodontitis has not been evaluated in detail. Due to these reasons, this study was designed to evaluate whether tonsillectomy significantly influenced CP. Based on these pivotal observations, we designed the present study to assess whether periodontal parameters significantly influenced serum vitamin D levels.

The purpose of this study was to compare the risk of CP between participants who underwent tonsillectomy and those who did not (control participants) using a national cohort dataset. It was hypothesized that tonsillectomy would decrease the risk of CP. In this study, those who underwent tonsillectomy and the control participants were matched using a 1:4 ratio, adjusting for age, sex, region of residence, pre-index date CP treatment, obesity, smoking, alcohol consumption, and Charlson comorbidity index (CCI) score.

2. Materials and Methods

2.1. Study Population

The ethics committee of Hallym University (2019-01-003) approved this study. Written informed consent was waived by the Institutional Review Board. All analyses adhered to the guidelines and regulations of the ethics committee of Hallym University. A detailed description of The Korean National Health Insurance Service-Health Screening Cohort data is given elsewhere [27].

2.2. Tonsillectomy

Tonsillectomy was defined using operation code Q2300.

2.3. Chronic Periodontitis

Patients with CP were diagnosed based on ICD-10 codes (K05.3) and were treated by dentists. The number of CP treatments was counted from the date of tonsillectomy treatment (index date [ID]) to the date before the two-year period (pre-ID CP for 2 y). The number of CP treatments was also counted from the index date to the date after the first-year period (post-ID 1 y CP, post-operative 1–365 days), second-year period (post-ID 2 y CP, post-operative 366–730 days), third-year period (post-ID 3 y CP, post-operative 731–1095 days), fourth-year period (post-ID 4 y CP, post-operative 1096–1460 days), and fifth-year period (post-ID 5 y CP, post-operative 1461–1825 days).

2.4. Participant Selection

Patients who underwent tonsillectomy were selected from 514,866 participants with 497,931,549 medical claim codes (n = 1321). A control group was included if participants had not undergone tonsillectomy between 2002 and 2015 (n = 513,545). To select tonsillectomy patients who were diagnosed for the first time, we excluded those who were diagnosed from 2002 to 2003 (washout periods, n = 228). Patients who underwent tonsillectomy were matched 1:4 with control participants based on age, sex, income, and region of residence. To analyze the subgroups according to pre-ID CP for 2 y, tonsillectomy patients were additionally matched with pre-ID CP for 2 y with a categorical variable (0 times, 1 time, and ≥2 times). To minimize the selection bias, the control participants were selected in random number order. The index date of each tonsillectomy patient was set as the time of the tonsillectomy treatment. The index date of control participants was set as the index date of their matched tonsillectomy. Therefore, each tonsillectomy patient that was subsequently matched with the control participants had the same index date. During the 1:4 matching process, 509,173 un-matched control participants were excluded. Participants who were recorded in 2015 were excluded to calculate post-ID 1 y CP (n = 49 for tonsillectomy patients, n = 196 for control participants). Finally, 1044 patients who underwent tonsillectomy were matched 1:4 with 4176 control participants; see Figure 1.

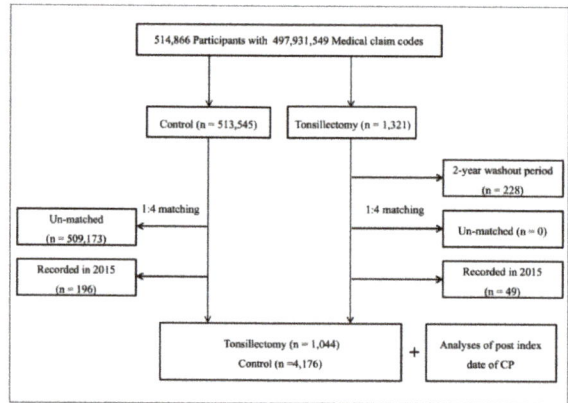

Figure 1. A schematic illustration of the participant selection process that was used in the present study. Of a total of 514,866 participants, 1044 of tonsillectomy participants were matched with 4176 control participants based on age, sex, income, region of residence, and pre-index date (ID) chronic periodontitis (CP) for 2 y.

2.5. Covariates

The age groups were divided by the following 5-year intervals: 40–44, 45–49, 50–54 ... , and 85+ years old. Income groups were organized into five classes (class 1 [lowest income] to 5 [highest income]). The region of residence was classed as either urban (Seoul, Busan, Daegu, Incheon, Gwangju, Daejeon, and Ulsan) or rural (Gyeonggi, Gangwon, Chungcheongbuk, Chungcheongnam, Jeollabuk, Jeollanam, Gyeongsangbuk, Gyeongsangnam, and Jeju).

Tobacco smoking was categorized based on the current smoking status of the participant (nonsmoker, past smoker, or current smoker). Alcohol consumption was categorized on the basis of the frequency of alcohol consumption (<1 time a week or ≥1 time a week). Obesity was measured using body mass index (BMI, kg/m^2). Missing BMI variables were replaced by mean BMI from final selected participants. BMI was categorized as <18.5 (underweight), ≥18.5 to <23 (normal), ≥23 to <25 (overweight), ≥25 to <30 (obese I), or ≥30 (obese II) based on the Asia-Pacific criteria following the Western Pacific Regional Office (WPRO) 2000.

The Charlson Comorbidity Index (CCI) has been widely used to measure disease burden using 17 comorbidities. A score was given to each participant depending on the severity and number of diseases they presented with. CCI was measured as a continuous variable (0 [no comorbidities] through 29 [multiple comorbidities]) [28]. The scores were calculated and the final CCI score was used as a covariate in the analyses.

2.6. Statistical Analyses

The general characteristics between the tonsillectomy and control groups were compared using a Chi-square test.

A simple linear regression and a multiple linear regression were used to calculate the estimated values and 95% of the confidence intervals (CI) for post-ID 1 y CP, post-ID 2 y CP, post-ID 3 y CP, post-ID 4 y CP, and post-ID 5 y CP in the tonsillectomy group compared to the control group. Both the simple linear regression and the multiple linear regression were stratified by age, sex, income, and region of residence. In the multiple linear regression, the model was adjusted for obesity, smoking status, alcohol consumption, CCI score, and pre-ID CP for 2 y as a continuous variable.

For the subgroup analyses, we divided participants by age (<60 years old and ≥60 years old), sex (male or female), and pre-ID CP for 2 y (0 times, 1 time, and ≥2 times) using a crude model and an adjusted model.

Two-tailed analyses were performed, and significance was defined as *p*-value less than 0.05. The SAS version 9.4 (SAS Institute Inc., Cary, NC, USA) was used for statistical analysis.

3. Results

Age, sex, income, and region of residence were matched between tonsillectomy and control participants exactly ($p = 1.000$), while obesity, smoking, and CCI were different ($p < 0.05$, Table 1). The number of CP treatments prior to the index date were matched as the categorical variable.

Table 1. General Characteristics of Participants.

Characteristics	Total Participants		
	Tonsillectomy (n, %)	Control (n, %)	*p*-Value
Age (years old)			1.000
40–44	74 (7.1)	296 (7.1)	
45–49	252 (24.1)	1008 (24.1)	
50–54	324 (31.0)	1296 (31.0)	
55–59	226 (21.7)	904 (21.7)	
60–64	100 (9.6)	400 (9.6)	
65–69	46 (4.4)	184 (4.4)	
70–74	13 (1.3)	52 (1.3)	
75–79	6 (0.6)	24 (0.6)	
80–84	3 (0.3)	12 (0.3)	
Sex			1.000
Male	720 (69.0)	2880 (69.0)	
Female	324 (31.0)	1296 (31.0)	
Income			1.000
1 (lowest)	114 (10.9)	456 (10.9)	
2	105 (10.1)	420 (10.1)	
3	127 (12.2)	508 (12.2)	
4	216 (20.7)	864 (20.7)	
5 (highest)	482 (46.2)	1928 (46.2)	
Region of residence			1.000
Urban	527 (50.5)	2108 (50.5)	
Rural	517 (49.5)	2068 (49.5)	
Pre index date of CP			1.000
0 time	701 (67.2)	2804 (67.2)	
1 time	145 (13.9)	580 (13.9)	
≥2 times	198 (19.0)	792 (19.0)	
Obesity [†]			<0.001 *
Underweight	6 (0.6)	61 (1.5)	
Normal	245 (23.5)	1436 (34.4)	
Overweight	286 (27.4)	1143 (27.4)	
Obese I	442 (42.3)	1427 (34.2)	
Obese II	65 (6.2)	109 (2.6)	
Smoking status			0.019 *
Nonsmoker	611 (58.5)	2483 (59.5)	
Past smoker	193 (18.5)	633 (15.2)	
Current smoker	240 (23.0)	1060 (25.4)	
Alcohol consumption			0.219
<1 time a week	647 (62.0)	2501 (59.9)	
≥1 time a week	397 (38.0)	1675 (40.1)	
CCI score			<0.001 *
0	713 (68.3)	3,275 (78.4)	
1	168 (16.1)	448 (10.7)	
2	85 (8.1)	240 (5.8)	
3	29 (2.8)	91 (2.2)	
≥4	49 (4.7)	122 (2.9)	

Abbreviations: CCI, Charlson comorbidity index; CP, chronic periodontitis. * Chi-square test. Significance at $p < 0.05$. [†] Obesity (BMI, body mass index, kg/m^2) was categorized as <18.5 (underweight), ≥18.5 to <23 (normal), ≥23 to <25 (overweight), ≥25 to <30 (obese I), and ≥30 (obese II).

The adjusted estimated value (EV) of the number of post-ID CP did not reach statistical significance in any post-ID year (each of $p > 0.05$, Table 2). In the subgroup analyses according to age and sex, statistical significance was only reached in ≥60-year-old men in post ID 2 y (EV = 0.561, 95% CI = 0.156–0.967, $p = 0.007$, Figure 2). In another subgroup analysis according to the number of pre-ID CP, statistical significance was not found in any analysis, see Figure 3.

Table 2. Simple and multiple linear regression model (estimated value [95% confidence interval]) for post-index date of CP (post-ID CP) periods in tonsillectomy group compared to control group.

Characteristics	Linear Regression			
	Simple [†]	p-Value	Multiple [†,‡]	p-Value
Post ID 1 y CP (n = 5220)				
Tonsillectomy	−0.068 (−0.153 to 0.018)	0.123	−0.073 (−0.158 to 0.012)	0.091
Post ID 2 y CP (n = 4920)				
Tonsillectomy	0.009 (−0.083 to 0.100)	0.853	0.021 (−0.069 to 0.111)	0.649
Post ID 3 y CP (n = 4610)				
Tonsillectomy	−0.055 (−0.163 to 0.052)	0.313	−0.040 (−0.148 to 0.067)	0.459
Post ID 4 y CP (n = 4245)				
Tonsillectomy	0.052 (−0.064 to 0.169)	0.377	0.059 (−0.058 to 0.176)	0.325
Post ID 5 y CP (n = 3825)				
Tonsillectomy	0.031 (−0.092 to 0.153)	0.623	0.054 (−0.069 to 0.177)	0.388

Abbreviations: CCI, Charlson comorbidity index; CP, chronic periodontitis. Linear regression model, Significance at $p < 0.05$. [†] Models stratified by age, sex, income, and region of residence. [‡] A model adjusted for obesity, smoking, alcohol consumption, CCI scores, and pre-index date of CP (pre-ID CP) for 2 y.

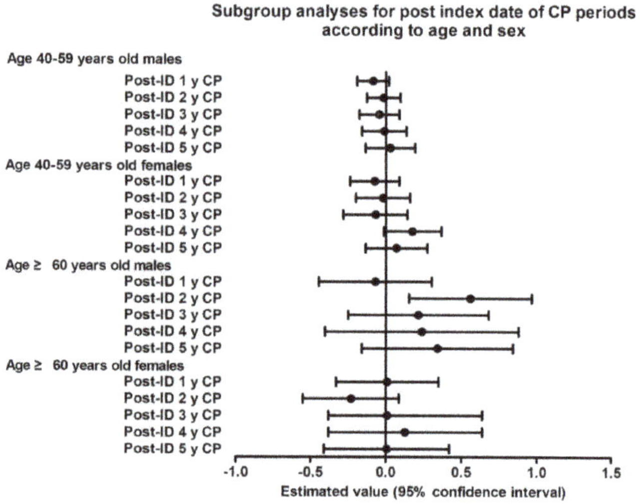

Figure 2. Subgroup analyses of simple and multiple linear regression models (estimated value [95% confidence interval]) for post-index date of CP (post-ID CP) periods in tonsillectomy group compared to control group according to age and sex.

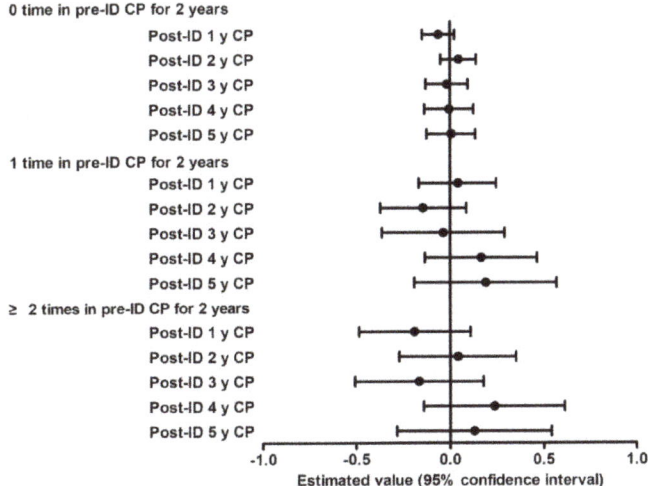

Figure 3. Subgroup analyses of simple and multiple linear regression models (estimated value [95% confidence interval]) for post-index date of CP (post-ID CP) periods in tonsillectomy and control groups according to pre-index date of CP (pre-ID CP) for 2 years.

4. Discussion

The hypothesis of this study, based on previous research that suggests a link between peritonsillar infection and periodontitis, was that the bacteriological and clinical outcomes of tonsillectomy could influence the diagnosis and treatment of CP [29]. It has previously been suggested that the niches around the palatine tonsils are the sources of bacterial infection for the periodontal area [18,23].

Unexpectedly, this study revealed that the adjusted EV of the number of post-ID CP did not reach statistical significance in any post-ID year. In another subgroup analysis according to the number of pre-ID CP, statistical significance was not found in any analysis. These findings oppose the assumption made by Quiryinen et al., although limitations of this study should be further discussed [18].

Tonsillectomy, including removal of the biofilm, has a positive effect on the intraoral areas such as the gingiva and tongue. A previous study reported that the microorganisms in the tongue area were altered following tonsillectomy [26]. The study showed that *Tannerella forsythia* and *Porphyromonas gingivalis* levels decreased in samples taken from the tongue after tonsillectomy [26]. This result could be explained by how anatomically close the tongue and tonsils are, and the fact that saliva is exchanged between them while speaking and swallowing. On the contrary, the same study reported that lesser changes occurred in other bacteria levels in the periodontal pocket following tonsillectomy [26]. They suggested that, with regards to the tonsillar area, the periodontal pocket would be more distant and difficult to access than the tongue area. As such, other bacteria in the periodontal pocket may be less affected. We also believe that the risk of developing CP after tonsillectomy was not reduced in our study for this reason.

Another reason for the discrepancy between the diagnosis and treatment of CP and tonsillectomy is that the major bacteria in culture-dependent studies of tonsils and the microbiome in culture-independent 16 s sequencing studies are *Streptococcus* and *Haemophilus influenzae* [8,30]. However, the essential microbiome in CP was *Porpyromonas gingivalis*, which can increase the activity of biofilm bacteria by interrupting homeostasis in the host.

Our findings could be explained by the improvements that occur with regards to mouth breathing following tonsillectomy. Tonsillectomy can eliminate breathing problems such as snoring or mouth breathing [31], which is likely to increase the risk of periodontitis. Kaur et al. have reported that a patient's periodontal condition is influenced by mouth breathing even after periodontal treatment such as scaling and root planning [32]. Mouth breathing also induces a dry condition in the intraoral area, which could increase the possibility of periodontitis. This hypothesis was explained in another study, suggesting that the salivary substitute had a positive effect on the periodontal condition in mouth breathing patients with CP [33]. According to these studies, tonsillectomy might reduce mouth breathing, and improved mouth breathing could have a beneficial effect on periodontitis.

This study has four advantages. The first is the large number of study participants (n = 5220). Participants were followed up for a maximum of 13 years following tonsillectomy, whereas a similar study only conducted a 3-year follow-up [29]. Secondly, the Korean National Health Insurance Service-Health Screening Cohort dataset is a large national survey that is representative of the Korean population. These cohort records were available for each participant, and the records used in our study were not distorted by the memory of participants. The data are also inclusive of all Koreans without exception; therefore, no participants were missed during the follow-up period. Thirdly, well-trained clinicians documented general health examinations and laboratory evaluations. Finally, adjusting factors showed a statistically significant independent association with tonsillectomy in our data, thus confirming the reliability of our study.

This study used a large population dataset; nevertheless, the findings have limitations. Firstly, the dataset included many factors such as alcohol consumption, obesity, smoking, and age. However, it was impossible to adjust for all systemic factors that were not included in the dataset. Secondly, this study could have been subject to surveillance bias. Tonsillectomy was more likely to be diagnosed for possibly unrelated CP, based on a higher number of visits to medical institutions. However, it is very unlikely that increased participant visits would induce the detection of CP. Dental examinations were conducted during regular visits that were covered by the Korean National Health Service (KNHS), which has exclusive characteristics, including low payment, widespread coverage, and easy access to medical institutions in Korea. In addition to these advantages, most Koreans undergo regular dental check-ups. Additionally, the large population dataset of this study was adjusted for many factors; thus, the surveillance bias was minimized by this adjustment. Therefore, this study prevented surveillance bias by adjusting the characteristics of the KNHS system. Furthermore, the present study analyzed the association using only code from data of the Korean National Health Service (KNHS), and thus the data did not indicate periodontitis severity. There may also be confounders that were not adjusted for. Finally, data were collected from individuals over the age of 40 years. Therefore, considering these limitations, further studies are required to validate our findings.

5. Conclusions

This study revealed that tonsillectomy was not significantly associated with reducing CP. Though the tonsils and periodontium are close in location, and tonsillectomy and CP may be related with regards to bacterial inflammation, the risk of CP in patients undergoing tonsillectomy was not statistically significant. However, further studies with a larger population should be considered to confirm, with greater plausibility, the influence of tonsillectomy on periodontal conditions in patients affected by CP.

Author Contributions: Conceptualization, S.H.B. and H.G.C.; Data curation, C.M. and H.G.C.; Formal analysis, B.J.P. and H.G.C.; Funding acquisition, S.J.H.; Investigation, S.H.B., H.K., S.H.K., B.J.P., and H.G.C.; Methodology, C.M., B.J.P., and H.G.C.; Resources, S.J.H.; Supervision, S.H.B., Y.B.K., and S.J.H.; Visualization, S.H.B. and J.H.W.; Writing—Original draft, S.H.B. and S.J.H.; Writing—Review and editing, S.H.B., H.K., and S.J.H. All authors have read and agreed to the published version of the manuscript.

Funding: This research was supported by Hallym University Research Fund 2016 (HURF-2016-25).

Conflicts of Interest: The authors declare no potential conflicts of interest with respect to the authorship and/or publication of this article.

References

1. Dentino, A.; Lee, S.; Mailhot, J.; Hefti, A.F. Principles of periodontology. *Periodontology 2000* **2013**, *61*, 16–53. [CrossRef] [PubMed]
2. Socransky, S.S. Microbiology of periodontal disease—Present status and future considerations. *J. Periodontol.* **1977**, *48*, 497–504. [CrossRef] [PubMed]
3. Stingu, C.S.; Jentsch, H.; Eick, S.; Schaumann, R.; Knofler, G.; Rodloff, A. Microbial profile of patients with periodontitis compared with healthy subjects. *Quintessence Int.* **2012**, *43*, e23–e31. [PubMed]
4. Socransky, S.S.; Haffajee, A.D.; Cugini, M.A.; Smith, C.; Kent, R.L., Jr. Microbial complexes in subgingival plaque. *J. Clin. Periodontol.* **1998**, *25*, 134–144. [CrossRef] [PubMed]
5. Persic Bukmir, R.; Jurcevic Grgic, M.; Brumini, G.; Spalj, S.; Pezelj-Ribaric, S.; Brekalo Prso, I. Influence of tobacco smoking on dental periapical condition in a sample of Croatian adults. *Wien. Klin. Wochenschr.* **2016**, *128*, 260–265. [CrossRef] [PubMed]
6. Dietrich, T.; Walter, C.; Oluwagbemigun, K.; Bergmann, M.; Pischon, T.; Pischon, N.; Boeing, H. Smoking, Smoking Cessation, and Risk of Tooth Loss: The EPIC-Potsdam Study. *J. Dent. Res.* **2015**, *94*, 1369–1375. [CrossRef]
7. Chavarry, N.G.; Vettore, M.V.; Sansone, C.; Sheiham, A. The relationship between diabetes mellitus and destructive periodontal disease: A meta-analysis. *Oral Health Prev. Dent.* **2009**, *7*, 107–127.
8. Jensen, A.; Fago-Olsen, H.; Sorensen, C.H.; Kilian, M. Molecular mapping to species level of the tonsillar crypt microbiota associated with health and recurrent tonsillitis. *PLoS ONE* **2013**, *8*, e56418. [CrossRef]
9. Kim, E.K.; Lee, S.G.; Choi, Y.H.; Won, K.C.; Moon, J.S.; Merchant, A.T.; Lee, H.-K. Association between diabetes-related factors and clinical periodontal parameters in type-2 diabetes mellitus. *BMC Oral Health* **2013**, *13*, 64. [CrossRef]
10. Nagasawa, Y.; Iio, K.; Fukuda, S.; Date, Y.; Iwatani, H.; Yamamoto, R.; Horii, A.; Inohara, H.; Imai, E.; Nakanishi, T.; et al. Periodontal disease bacteria specific to tonsil in IgA nephropathy patients predicts the remission by the treatment. *PLoS ONE* **2014**, *9*, e81636. [CrossRef]
11. Isola, G.; Matarese, G.; Ramaglia, L.; Pedulla, E.; Rapisarda, E.; Iorio-Siciliano, V. Association between periodontitis and glycosylated haemoglobin before diabetes onset: A cross-sectional study. *Clin. Oral Investig.* **2019**. [CrossRef] [PubMed]
12. Isola, G.; Alibrandi, A.; Curro, M.; Matarese, M.; Ricca, S.; Matarese, G.; Ientile, R.; Kocher, T. Evaluation of salivary and serum ADMA levels in patients with periodontal and cardiovascular disease as subclinical marker of cardiovascular risk. *J. Periodontol.* **2020**. [CrossRef] [PubMed]
13. Isola, G.; Alibrandi, A.; Rapisarda, E.; Matarese, G.; Williams, R.C.; Leonardi, R. Association of vitamin D in patients with periodontitis: A cross-sectional study. *J. Periodontal Res.* **2020**. [CrossRef]
14. Isola, G. Current Evidence of Natural Agents in Oral and Periodontal Health. *Nutrients* **2020**, *12*, 585. [CrossRef] [PubMed]
15. Slots, J. Low-cost periodontal therapy. *Periodontology 2000* **2012**, *60*, 110–137. [CrossRef] [PubMed]
16. Ramseier, C.A.; Warnakulasuriya, S.; Needleman, I.G.; Gallagher, J.E.; Lahtinen, A.; Ainamo, A.; Alajbeg, I.; Albert, D.; Al-Hazmi, N.; Antohe, M.E.; et al. Consensus Report: 2nd European Workshop on Tobacco Use Prevention and Cessation for Oral Health Professionals. *Int. Dent. J.* **2010**, *60*, 3–6. [PubMed]
17. Sahrmann, P.; Puhan, M.A.; Attin, T.; Schmidlin, P.R. Systematic review on the effect of rinsing with povidone-iodine during nonsurgical periodontal therapy. *J. Periodontal Res.* **2010**, *45*, 153–164. [CrossRef]
18. Quirynen, M.; Bollen, C.M.; Vandekerckhove, B.N.; Dekeyser, C.; Papaioannou, W.; Eyssen, H. Full- vs. partial-mouth disinfection in the treatment of periodontal infections: Short-term clinical and microbiological observations. *J. Dent. Res.* **1995**, *74*, 1459–1467. [CrossRef]
19. Mitchell, R.B.; Archer, S.M.; Ishman, S.L.; Rosenfeld, R.M.; Coles, S.; Finestone, S.A.; Friedman, N.R.; Giordano, T.; Hildrew, D.M.; Kim, T.W.; et al. Clinical Practice Guideline: Tonsillectomy in Children (Update). *Otolaryngol. Head Neck Surg.* **2019**, *160* (Suppl. 1), S1–S42. [CrossRef]
20. Bitar, M.A.; Dowli, A.; Mourad, M. The effect of tonsillectomy on the immune system: A systematic review and meta-analysis. *Int. J. Pediatr. Otorhinolaryngol.* **2015**, *79*, 1184–1191. [CrossRef]
21. Ingram, D.G.; Friedman, N.R. Toward Adenotonsillectomy in Children: A Review for the General Pediatrician. *JAMA Pediatr.* **2015**, *169*, 1155–1161. [CrossRef] [PubMed]

22. Quirynen, M.; De Soete, M.; Dierickx, K.; van Steenberghe, D. The intra-oral translocation of periodontopathogens jeopardises the outcome of periodontal therapy. A review of the literature. *J. Clin. Periodontol.* **2001**, *28*, 499–507. [CrossRef] [PubMed]
23. Cieplik, F.; Zaura, E.; Brandt, B.W.; Buijs, M.J.; Buchalla, W.; Crielaard, W.; Laine, M.L.; Deng, D.M.; Exterkate, R.A.M. Microcosm biofilms cultured from different oral niches in periodontitis patients. *J. Oral Microbiol.* **2019**, *11*, 1551596. [CrossRef] [PubMed]
24. Sakalauskiene, J.; Kubilius, R.; Gleiznys, A.; Vitkauskiene, A.; Ivanauskiene, E.; Saferis, V. Relationship of clinical and microbiological variables in patients with type 1 diabetes mellitus and periodontitis. *Med. Sci. Monit.* **2014**, *20*, 1871–1877. [CrossRef]
25. Develioglu, O.N.; Ipek, H.D.; Bahar, H.; Can, G.; Kulekci, M.; Aygun, G. Bacteriological evaluation of tonsillar microbial flora according to age and tonsillar size in recurrent tonsillitis. *Eur. Arch. Otorhinolaryngol.* **2014**, *271*, 1661–1665. [CrossRef]
26. Diener, V.N.; Gay, A.; Soyka, M.B.; Attin, T.; Schmidlin, P.R.; Sahrmann, P. What is the influence of tonsillectomy on the level of periodontal pathogens on the tongue dorsum and in periodontal pockets. *BMC Oral Health* **2018**, *18*, 62. [CrossRef]
27. Kim, S.Y.; Min, C.; Oh, D.J.; Choi, H.G. Tobacco Smoking and Alcohol Consumption Are Related to Benign Parotid Tumor: A Nested Case-Control Study Using a National Health Screening Cohort. *Clin. Exp. Otorhinolaryngol.* **2019**, *12*, 412–419. [CrossRef]
28. Quan, H.; Li, B.; Couris, C.M.; Fushimi, K.; Graham, P.; Hider, P.; Januel, J.-M.; Sundararajan, V. Updating and validating the Charlson comorbidity index and score for risk adjustment in hospital discharge abstracts using data from 6 countries. *Am. J. Epidemiol.* **2011**, *173*, 676–682. [CrossRef]
29. Georgalas, C.; Kanagalingam, J.; Zainal, A.; Ahmed, H.; Singh, A.; Patel, K.S. The association between periodontal disease and peritonsillar infection: A prospective study. *Otolaryngol. Head Neck Surg.* **2002**, *126*, 91–94. [CrossRef]
30. Liu, C.M.; Cosetti, M.K.; Aziz, M.; Buchhagen, J.L.; Contente-Cuomo, T.L.; Price, L.B.; Keim, P.S.; Lalwani, A.K. The otologic microbiome: A study of the bacterial microbiota in a pediatric patient with chronic serous otitis media using 16SrRNA gene-based pyrosequencing. *Arch. Otolaryngol. Head Neck Surg.* **2011**, *137*, 664–668. [CrossRef]
31. Zhang, L.Y.; Zhong, L.; David, M.; Cervin, A. Tonsillectomy or tonsillotomy? A systematic review for paediatric sleep-disordered breathing. *Int. J. Pediatr. Otorhinolaryngol.* **2017**, *103*, 41–50. [CrossRef] [PubMed]
32. Kaur, M.; Sharma, R.K.; Tewari, S.; Narula, S.C. Influence of mouth breathing on outcome of scaling and root planing in chronic periodontitis. *BDJ Open* **2018**, *4*, 17039. [CrossRef] [PubMed]
33. Bhatia, A.; Sharma, R.K.; Tewari, S.; Narula, S.C. A randomized clinical trial of salivary substitute as an adjunct to scaling and root planing for management of periodontal inflammation in mouth breathing patients. *J. Oral Sci.* **2015**, *57*, 241–247. [CrossRef] [PubMed]

© 2020 by the authors. Licensee MDPI, Basel, Switzerland. This article is an open access article distributed under the terms and conditions of the Creative Commons Attribution (CC BY) license (http://creativecommons.org/licenses/by/4.0/).

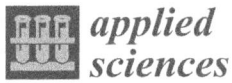

Article

Sex Prediction Based on Mesiodistal Width Data in the Portuguese Population

João Albernaz Neves [1], Nathalie Antunes-Ferreira [2,3], Vanessa Machado [1,4], João Botelho [1,4,*], Luís Proença [5], Alexandre Quintas [2,3], José João Mendes [1,4] and Ana Sintra Delgado [1,4]

1. Clinical Research Unit (CRU), Centro de Investigação Interdisciplinar Egas Moniz (CiiEM), Egas Moniz, CRL, 2829-511 Caparica, Almada, Portugal; jalbernazneves@gmail.com (J.A.N.); vanessamachado558@gmail.com (V.M.); jmendes@egasmoniz.edu.pt (J.J.M.); anasintradelgado@gmail.com (A.S.D.)
2. Laboratório de Ciências Forenses e Psicológicas Egas Moniz (LCFPEM), Centro de Investigação Interdisciplinar Egas Moniz (CiiEM), Egas Moniz CRL, 2829-511 Caparica, Almada, Portugal; natantfer@gmail.com (N.A.-F.); alexandre.quintas@gmail.com (A.Q.)
3. Laboratory of Biological Anthropology and Human Osteology (LABOH), CRIA/FCSH, Universidade NOVA de Lisboa, 1069-061 Lisboa, Portugal
4. Orthodontics Department, Egas Moniz Dental Clinic (EMDC), Egas Moniz, CRL, 2829-511 Caparica, Almada, Portugal
5. Quantitative Methods for Health Research (MQIS), CiiEM, Egas Moniz, CRL, 2829-511 Caparica, Almada, Portugal; lproenca@egasmoniz.edu.pt
* Correspondence: jbotelho@egasmoniz.edu.pt; Tel.: +351-21-294-6700

Received: 21 May 2020; Accepted: 13 June 2020; Published: 17 June 2020

Abstract: Accurate sex prediction is a key step in creating a postmortem forensic profile as it excludes approximately half the population. It is our goal to develop a predictive model to establish sex through teeth mesiodistal widths in a Portuguese population. The pretreatment dental casts of 168 of Portuguese orthodontics subjects (59 males and 109 females) were included. Mesiodistal widths from right first molar to left first molar were measured on each pretreatment cast to the nearest 0.01 mm using a digital caliper. Overall, the mesiodistal widths of the upper and lower canines, premolars, and molars were found to be significantly different between females and males. Conversely, no significant differences between sexes were identified for incisors. A multivariate logistic regression model for sex prediction was developed and the teeth included in the final reduced model being the upper left canine (2.3), the lower right lateral incisor (4.2) and the lower right canine (4.3). There is a prevalence of sexual dimorphism in all teeth except the incisors. The canines present the most noticeable difference between sexes. The presented sex determination predictive model exhibits an overall correct classification of 75%, outperforming all available models for this purpose and therefore is a potential tool for forensic analysis in this population.

Keywords: forensic dentistry; sex determination; sexual dimorphism; dental measurements; predictive model; Portuguese population

1. Introduction

Forensic dentistry emerges as a part of forensic medicine and dental anthropology. This is the branch of dentistry that focuses on the issues of identifying human remains by direct comparison, bite mark identification, clinical malpractice, and forensic dental profiling, such as sex and age estimation, in cases of unknown human remains, in order to facilitate their subsequent identification [1,2].

Teeth are the hardest organ in the human body and very important in postmortem identification procedures. Although pelvic and cranial bones can be more accurate in identifying sex, they are rarely in optimal condition in extreme cases, such as natural disasters or mass graves, which may prevent accurate estimation through them. Teeth are considered quite useful in these scenarios as they are often recovered intact [3–6]. However, there may be some setbacks that prevent dental eruption of teeth useful for forensic identification [7–10].

Accurate sex prediction is a key step in creating a postmortem forensic profile as it excludes approximately half the population [11]. Several studies state that teeth have a high degree of sexual dimorphism [2,4,5,12,13]. Generally, male teeth are larger than female teeth, however data are not consensual and reverse dimorphism also occurs [4,12]. Sexual dimorphism may vary between different populations, possibly due to variations in the environment, available food resources, or genetic pool [3,14].

The most usual way to obtain data is from dental casts using a digital caliper. There are several measures to take into account and their analysis may be performed through direct comparison of measures, statistical analyses, or indexes.

Only two previous studies presented potential predictive sex models for Portuguese populations using dental measurements. Pereira et al. (2010) [1], using upper canine-to-canine teeth, rendered a combination of incisors mesiodistal and canine diagonal distances. As the proposed model was confined to only six teeth, it lacks a complete teeth analysis. On the other hand, Silva et al. (2015) [12] employed the mandibular canine index [15] with a modest success rate of 64.2%, concluding that this index should be restrictively applied to the Portuguese scenario in sex identification.

Given the lack of robust sex identification models for the Portuguese population, we aimed to use cast models of a previously studied sample (Machado et al., 2018) [16] to develop a new sex prediction model based on mesiodistal width measures. We hypothesize that there is a sex-based teeth dimorphism in this population and it is distinguishable through a predictive model; therefore our null hypothesis is that such dimorphism may not exist.

2. Materials and Methods

2.1. Study Design

This study used a previously reported sample [16] that has received approval by the Egas Moniz Ethics Committee (Number 600). Written informed consents were obtained from all participants during their first appointment at the Orthodontic Department of the Egas Moniz Dental Clinic.

This investigation follows the transparent reporting of a multivariable prediction model for individual prognosis or diagnosis (TRIPOD) reporting guidelines [17] for validation of prediction models (see supplementary material). This study was conducted on a triple-blind basis with respect to diagnosis and clinical outcome, data collection, and analysis.

2.2. Participants

The assessment tool consisted of pre-treatment dental casts, a part of standard orthodontic treatment planning, in dental stone selected from the archives of the Egas Moniz Dental Clinic Orthodontic Department (Almada, Portugal). From a total of 541 casts gathered from November 2010 to December 2017, 168 (59 males and 109 females) were selected according to the inclusion and exclusion criteria.

The inclusion criteria were: all teeth, from first molar in the right side to first molar in the left side in both upper and lower jaws, were fully erupted and present; no history of interproximal stripping; no proximal caries that might interfere with precise tooth measurement; no restorations, abrasions or attrition; no previous or ongoing orthodontic treatment; no abnormal tooth morphology or congenitally missing or impacted [16]. All patients failing to fulfil these criteria were excluded.

2.3. Dental Casts Analysis and Measurement Reproducibility

Dental cast measurements were performed by one researcher (VM) using a digital caliper to measure the mesiodistal tooth widths from the right first molar to the left first molar to the nearest 0.01 mm. The mesiodistal width of each tooth was measured at the widest distance between the mesial and distal contact points. The position of the caliper had to be perpendicular to the occlusal surface of the measured tooth [1,11,14,16,18–21].

Ten study casts were randomly chosen from the total of 168 and remeasured one week later by the same investigator (V.M.). Intraclass correlation coefficient (ICC) was calculated with an absolute agreement of ICC = 0.98.

2.4. Statistical Analysis

Data analysis was performed using IBM SPSS Statistics version 25.0 for Windows (Armonk, NY: IBM Corp.). Descriptive statistics as mean and standard deviation (SD) were determined for the mesiodistal width per tooth. Mean mesiodistal width for each tooth was compared according to sex and by Student's t-test. A multivariate stepwise adjusted logistic regression procedure was applied to derive a reduced predictive model for sex determination based on the mesiodistal widths for each tooth. To test the performance of the obtained model and compare it to previous ones, the sensitivity, specificity, accuracy, and precision were determined for all models when applied to the studied sample [22]. Performance measurement was assessed by binary area under the curve (AUC) and through receiver operating characteristics (ROC) analysis. The level of significance was set at 5%, in all statistical inference analyses.

3. Results

3.1. Mesiodistal Width Per Tooth

In the studied sample the mean age was 20.1 (±7.3) (see Machado et al., 2018 [16] for a detailed description). The mean mesiodistal width for each tooth, according to sex, is presented in Table 1. Overall, the mean mesiodistal widths of upper and lower canines, premolars, and molars were found to be significantly different between females and males. Regarding the incisors, no significant differences were found as a function of sex.

Table 1. Descriptive values of mesiodistal width (mm), presented as mean and standard deviation (SD) for each tooth, as a function of sex (n = 168).

Semi-Arch	Tooth Type	Tooth Code	Female (n = 109)		Male (n = 59)		p-Value *
			Mean (±SD)	Range (Min–Max)	Mean (±SD)	Range (Min–Max)	
Upper right	Molar	1.6	10.13 (±0.56)	8.50–12.52	10.40 (±0.60)	9.26–12.37	**0.004**
	Premolars	1.5	6.62 (±0.47)	5.51–8.04	6.40 (±0.52)	5.71–8.30	**0.008**
		1.4	6.93 (±0.47)	5.70–8.17	7.18 (±0.48)	6.35–8.50	**0.001**
	Canine	1.3	7.67 (±0.46)	6.40–8.90	7.97 (±0.57)	6.10–9.22	**<0.001**
	Incisors	1.2	6.64 (±0.61)	5.20–7.89	6.70 (±0.63)	5.25–8.55	0.565
		1.1	8.60 (±0.58)	7.00–10.05	8.68 (±0.66)	6.47–10.78	0.414
Upper left	Incisors	2.1	8.62 (±0.54)	7.39–9.88	8.69 (±0.67)	6.47–10.66	0.437
		2.2	6.54 (±0.60)	4.73–7.89	6.71 (±0.65)	5.25–8.30	0.091
	Canine	2.3	7.65 (±0.46)	6.40–8.70	8.04 (±0.52)	6.83–9.22	**<0.001**
	Premolars	2.4	6.92 (±0.48)	5.70–8.17	7.17 (±0.50)	5.96–8.28	**0.002**
		2.5	6.62 (±0.47)	5.51–8.04	6.84 (±0.52)	5.70–8.30	**0.005**
	Molar	2.6	10.12 (±0.56)	8.50–12.52	10.33 (±0.59)	9.4–12.44	**0.018**
Lower right	Molar	4.6	10.63 (±0.61)	9.10–12.32	11.03 (±0.57)	9.82–12.17	**<0.001**
	Premolars	4.5	7.19 (±0.52)	6.04–8.93	7.36 (±0.54)	6.17–8.98	**0.050**
		4.4	7.08 (±0.43)	6.11–8.30	7.36 (±0.51)	6.22–8.50	**0.001**
	Canine	4.3	6.63 (±0.42)	5.84–8.15	7.01 (±0.48)	6.03–8.91	**<0.001**
	Incisors	4.2	5.89 (±0.43)	4.50–6.94	5.97 (±0.44)	4.98–6.95	0.253
		4.1	5.38 (±0.43)	4.50–7.60	5.46 (±0.43)	4.68–6.51	0.280
Lower left	Incisors	3.1	5.38 (±0.44)	4.50–7.60	5.41 (±0.47)	3.73–6.37	0.708
		3.2	5.86 (±0.44)	4.50–6.78	5.99 (±0.42)	4.92–6.99	0.052
	Canine	3.3	6.63 (±0.41)	5.84–8.16	7.00 (±0.50)	6.14–8.95	**<0.001**
	Premolars	3.4	7.03 (±0.50)	5.65–8.30	7.35 (±0.52)	6.22–8.50	**<0.001**
		3.5	7.14 (±0.50)	6.04–8.70	7.37 (±0.58)	6.00–8.98	**0.008**
	Molar	3.6	10.62 (±0.57)	9.10–12.32	11.00 (±0.61)	9.76–12.17	**<0.001**

Note: * Student's t-test. Significant p-values ($p < 0.05$) denoted in bold.

3.2. Sex Prediction Model Development

In order to develop a model for sex prediction based on the teeth mesiodistal width, a multivariate logistic regression procedure was implemented considering a first stage that included all teeth that exhibited significant differences in the sex-based comparison: canines, premolars and molars. Then, a stepwise adjusted logistic regression procedure derived a reduced best fitting model that is depicted in Table 2. In this final optimized model, the upper left canine (2.3), the lower right lateral incisor (4.2) and the lower right canine (4.3) were the only teeth included.

Table 2. Final reduced logistic regression model (n = 168).

Variables	B	p-Value	EXP (B)	EXP (B) 95% CI	
				Lower	Upper
Tooth 2.3	1.208	0.019	3.35	1.22	9.22
Tooth 4.3	1.800	0.003	6.05	1.84	19.91
Tooth 4.2	−1.317	0.018	0.27	0.09	0.80
Constant	−14.546	<0.001	-	-	-

$R^2(N)$ = 0.268, % correct classification = 75%; H&L: X^2 = 6.767 (p = 0.562); Note: outcome variable (sex) coded as male: 1, female: 0.

From the fitted model data, the following formula can be derived:

$$\ln(p/(1-p)) = -14.546 + 1.208x + 1.800y - 1.317z$$

where p is the probability of an individual being classified as male, with a lower cutoff value of 0.5, and with x, y, and z representing the mesiodistal width of the upper left canine (2.3), lower right canine (4.3) and lower right lateral incisor (4.2), respectively.

3.3. Comparison with Previous Models

The achieved model was then compared to the previous sex prediction tools by means of performance when applied to this sample (Table 3).

Table 3. Performance assessment of the different models when applied to the studied sample. Measures are presented as percentage. For AUC, estimation by a 95% confidence interval (95% CI) is also shown.

Model		Sensitivity (%)	Specificity (%)	Accuracy (%)	Precision (%)	AUC within ROC Analysis (95% CI)
Acharya et al., 2007 [23]	Model 1	85.3	50.8	73.2	76.2	0.642 (0.551–0.733)
	Model 2	13.8	93.2	41.7	78.9	0.637 (0.546–0.728)
Mitsea et al., 2014 [4]		65.1	45.8	58.3	68.9	0.681 (0.592–0.770)
Peckmann et al., 2016 [5]	Model 1	89.9	39.0	72.0	73.1	0.535 (0.445–0.625)
	Model 2	59.6	49.2	56.0	68.4	0.555 (0.463–0.646)
	Model 3	65.1	45.8	58.3	68.9	0.644 (0.553–0.736)
	Model 4	88.1	37.3	70.2	72.2	0.544 (0.452–0.636)
	Model 5	86.2	37.3	69.0	71.8	0.555 (0.463–0.646)
	Model 6	82.6	45.8	69.6	73.8	0.627 (0.535–0.719)
	Model 7	81.7	45.8	69.0	73.6	0.618 (0.525–0.710)
Neves et al., 2020		87.2	52.5	75.0	77.2	0.768 (0.693–0.843)

AUC—Area under the curve; ROC—Receiver operating characteristic.

4. Discussion

Sex estimation is a vital step in forensic medicine for body identification both in single and mass disaster events. In the Portuguese scenario, sex estimation models through dental hard tissues are scarce and previous proposed models lacked consistency and only accounted for a small subset of teeth. Therefore, we aimed to develop a potential model using mesiodistal widths of models cast previously for studies of orthodontic indexes. Then, we compared the performance of this model with other full-mouth mesiodistal models published elsewhere. Overall, our model outperformed all available strategies and might be used as a forensic tool for sex estimation in Portuguese samples.

As previously stated, sexual dimorphism may vary between populations, possibly due to a variety of reasons [3,14]. Therefore, this new model arises as a valuable tool to forensic dentistry.

Our results have prospective importance. (1) Until now, there were no models developed for the Portuguese population from complete models. (2) Dental hard tissues are of utmost interest because they are the most lasting tissue of human body, even in post-mortem difficult conditions. (3) This tool may be very useful in single or mass disasters or body identification cases in Portugal, especially due to the unpredictability of these situations. (4) These results confirm sexual dimorphism on teeth mesiodistal width in canines, premolars, and molars of the upper and lower arches.

Dental crown dimensions can be obtained through intraoral measurements [18], dental forms [4,11,13,14,16,19,24], or human remains [20,21]. The mesiodistal and buccolingual measurements of the crown were the two most commonly used and studied dimensions [1,11,14,18–21], followed by diagonal measurements (mesiobuccal-distolingual and distobuccal-mesiolingual) [1,21,25] and the canine mandibular index (expressed as the ratio between the mesiodistal dimension of the canines and the width of the intercanine arch [12,15,19,26]). These studies have shown that canine dimensions provide the highest sexual dimorphism [16,18,21,24,25], followed by premolars [21,25], first and second molars [20,21,25,27].

In this study, we analyzed the degree of sexual dimorphism in different teeth by measuring the maximum mesiodistal diameters of fully erupted permanent teeth from study casts. Overall, several teeth are sexually dimorphic and the crown mesiodistal dimensions were larger on average in males than in females. The results of this study confirm what was previously demonstrated, canine teeth are the most dimorphic teeth [1–5,7,19,21,24–26] but also molars present significant differences between sexes [11,13,23,25,28–30]. Within the elements that fit into our sex prediction model, the upper left canine, the lower right lateral incisor, and the lower right canine were the most appropriate and with better replicability.

Regarding the performance, our developed model outperformed previous published indexes in terms of AUC. In terms of accuracy and precision values, our model also outperformed the remaining models (75.0% and 77.2% for accuracy and precision, respectively). Furthermore, for sensitivity and specificity, this newly developed model presented the best combination of results, only being outperformed in sensitivity by Peckmann et al., 2016 [5] (model 4) and in specificity by Acharya et al., 2007 [23] (model 2).

Like other methodologies used in sex prediction, the amount and quality of evidence available for analysis are critical in forensic investigation. Some limitations of the applied methodology include any post-eruptive changes such as caries, interproximal wear, and interproximal restorations, which compromises the correct measurement of the teeth.

5. Strengths and Limitations

A possible limitation of this study is the fact that we have not accounted for second molars, mainly because the data that this analysis is derived from is an orthodontic population whose main purpose was to study a mesiodistal proportion measure. This measure, Bolton's analysis [31], only accounts for the mesiodistal width from the first molar to the first molar. Nevertheless, two previous large-base studies from this population revealed that second molars are one of the most commonly missing teeth, aside from first molars and premolars [32,33]. Interestingly, none of them accounted for the final model. Another possible limitation is the fact that the new model emerged from the same sample being studied, which may influence the results. The new model should be further investigated with a new sample in a future study.

6. Conclusions

Considering the limitations of this study, the present study found that there is a prevalence of sexual dimorphism in all teeth except the incisors and that the canines exhibit the most noticeable difference between sexes, followed by the first mandibular molars and premolars.

Through a stepwise adjusted logistic regression procedure, a suitable model for sex determination was developed. The reduced model was based on the upper left canine (2.3), the lower right lateral incisor (4.2), and the lower right canine (4.3) and achieved an accuracy of 75%.

Supplementary Materials: The following are available online at http://www.mdpi.com/2076-3417/10/12/4156/s1.

Author Contributions: Conceptualization, V.M. and J.B.; methodology, J.A.N.; validation, J.B., V.M. and L.P.; formal analysis, L.P.; investigation, J.A.N.; resources, A.S.D.; writing—original draft preparation, J.A.N.; writing—review and editing, J.J.M., N.A.-F. and A.Q.; supervision, J.J.M., A.S.D., N.A.-F. and A.Q.; project administration, J.J.M. and A.S.D. All authors have read and agreed to the published version of the manuscript.

Funding: This research received no external funding.

Conflicts of Interest: The authors declare no conflict of interest.

References

1. Pereira, C.; Bernardo, M.; Pestana, D.; Santos, J.C.; de Mendonça, M.C. Contribution of teeth in human forensic identification—Discriminant function sexing odontometrical techniques in Portuguese population. *J. Forensic Leg. Med.* **2010**, *17*, 105–110. [CrossRef]
2. Khamis, M.F.; Taylor, J.A.; Malik, S.N.; Townsend, G.C. Odontometric sex variation in Malaysians with application to sex prediction. *Forensic Sci. Int.* **2014**, *234*, 183.e1–183.e7. [CrossRef]
3. Işcan, M.Y.; Kedici, P.S. Sexual variation in bucco-lingual dimensions in Turkish dentition. *Forensic Sci. Int.* **2003**, *137*, 160–164. [CrossRef]
4. Mitsea, A.G.; Moraitis, K.; Leon, G.; Nicopoulou-Karayianni, K.; Spiliopoulou, C. Sex determination by tooth size in a sample of Greek population. *HOMO-J. Comp. Hum. Biol.* **2014**, *65*, 322–329. [CrossRef] [PubMed]
5. Peckmann, T.R.; Logar, C.; Garrido-Varas, C.E.; Meek, S.; Pinto, X.T. Sex determination using the mesio-distal dimension of permanent maxillary incisors and canines in a modern Chilean population. *Sci. Justice* **2016**, *56*, 84–89. [CrossRef] [PubMed]
6. Capitaneanu, C.; Willems, G.; Thevissen, P. A systematic review of odontological sex estimation methods. *J. Forensic Odontostomatol.* **2017**, *35*, 1–19. [PubMed]
7. Isola, G.; Anastasi, G.; Matarese, G.; Williams, R.; Cutroneo, G.; Bracco, P.; Piancino, M. Functional and molecular outcomes of the human masticatory muscles. *Oral Dis.* **2018**, *24*, 1428–1441. [CrossRef]
8. Isola, G.; Alibrandi, A.; Rapisarda, E.; Matarese, G.; Williams, R.C.; Leonardi, R. Association of vitamin D in patients with periodontitis: A cross-sectional study. *J. Periodontal Res.* **2020**, 1–11. [CrossRef]
9. Staderini, E.; Patini, R.; Guglielmi, F.; Camodeca, A.; Gallenzi, P. How to manage impacted third molars: Germectomy or delayed removal? A systematic literature review. *Medicina* **2019**, *55*, 79. [CrossRef]
10. Botelho, J.; Machado, V.; Proença, L.; Delgado, A.S.; Mendes, J.J. Vitamin D deficiency and oral health: A comprehensive review. *Nutrients* **2020**, *12*, 1471. [CrossRef]
11. Angadi, P.V.; Hemani, S.; Prabhu, S.; Acharya, A.B. Analyses of odontometric sexual dimorphism and sex assessment accuracy on a large sample. *J. Forensic Leg. Med.* **2013**, *20*, 673–677. [CrossRef] [PubMed]
12. Silva, A.M.; Pereira, M.L.; Gouveia, S.; Tavares, J.N.; Azevedo, Á.; Caldas, I.M. A new approach to sex estimation using the mandibular canine index. *Med. Sci. Law.* **2016**, *56*, 7–12. [CrossRef] [PubMed]
13. Prabhu, S.; Acharya, A.B. Odontometric sex assessment in Indians. *Forensic Sci. Int.* **2009**, *192*, 129.e1–129.e5. [CrossRef] [PubMed]
14. Brook, A.H.; Griffin, R.C.; Townsend, G.; Levisianos, Y.; Russell, J.; Smith, R.N. Variability and patterning in permanent tooth size of four human ethnic groups. *Arch. Oral Biol.* **2009**, *54*, 79–85. [CrossRef] [PubMed]
15. Rao, N.G.; Rao, N.N.; Pai, M.L.; Kotian, M.S. Mandibular canine index—A clue for establishing sex identity. *Forensic Sci. Int.* **1989**, *42*, 249–254. [CrossRef]
16. Machado, V.; Botelho, J.; Pereira, D.; Vasques, M.; Fernandes-Retto, P.; Proença, L.; Mendes, J.J.; Delgado, A. Bolton ratios in Portuguese subjects among different malocclusion groups. *J. Clin. Exp. Dent.* **2018**, *10*, e864–e868. [CrossRef]
17. Moons, K.G.M.; Altman, D.G.; Reitsma, J.B.; Ioannidis, J.P.A.; Macaskill, P.; Steyerberg, E.W.; Vickers, A.J.; Ransohoff, D.F.; Collins, G.S. Transparent reporting of a multivariable prediction model for individual prognosis or diagnosis (TRIPOD): Explanation and elaboration. *Ann. Intern. Med.* **2015**, *162*, W1–W73. [CrossRef] [PubMed]

18. Khangura, R.; Sircar, K.; Singh, S.; Rastogi, V. Sex determination using mesiodistal dimension of permanent maxillary incisors and canines. *J. Forensic Dent. Sci.* **2012**, *3*, 81. [CrossRef]
19. Phulari, R.S.; Rathore, R.; Talegaon, T.; Jariwala, P. Comparative assessment of maxillary canine index and maxillary first molar dimensions for sex determination in forensic odontology. *J. Forensic Dent. Sci.* **2017**, *9*, 110. [CrossRef]
20. Zorba, E.; Moraitis, K.; Manolis, S.K. Sexual dimorphism in permanent teeth of modern Greeks. *Forensic Sci. Int.* **2011**, *210*, 74–81. [CrossRef]
21. Zorba, E.; Moraitis, K.; Eliopoulos, C.; Spiliopoulou, C. Sex determination in modern Greeks using diagonal measurements of molar teeth. *Forensic Sci. Int.* **2012**, *217*, 19–26. [CrossRef] [PubMed]
22. Glas, A.S.; Lijmer, J.G.; Prins, M.H.; Bonsel, G.J.; Bossuyt, P.M.M. The diagnostic odds ratio: A single indicator of test performance. *J. Clin. Epidemiol.* **2003**, *56*, 1129–1135. [CrossRef]
23. Acharya, A.B.; Mainali, S. Univariate sex dimorphism in the Nepalese dentition and the use of discriminant functions in gender assessment. *Forensic Sci. Int.* **2007**, *173*, 47–56. [CrossRef] [PubMed]
24. Mujib, A.B.R.; Tarigoppula, R.K.V.N.; Kulkarni, P.G. Gender determination using diagonal measurements of maxillary molar and canine teeth in davangere population. *J. Clin. Diagn. Res.* **2014**, *8*, 141–144. [CrossRef]
25. Viciano, J.; López-Lázaro, S.; Alemán, I. Sex estimation based on deciduous and permanent dentition in a contemporary spanish population. *Am. J. Phys. Anthropol.* **2013**, *152*, 31–43. [CrossRef]
26. Acharya, A.B.; Angadi, P.V.; Prabhu, S.; Nagnur, S. Validity of the mandibular canine index (MCI) in sex prediction: Reassessment in an Indian sample. *Forensic Sci. Int.* **2011**, *204*, 207.e1–207.e4. [CrossRef]
27. Acharya, A.B.; Prabhu, S.; Muddapur, M.V. Odontometric sex assessment from logistic regression analysis. *Int. J. Leg. Med.* **2011**, *125*, 199–204. [CrossRef]
28. Thapar, R.; Angadi, P.V.; Hallikerimath, S.; Kale, A.D. Sex assessment using odontometry and cranial anthropometry: Evaluation in an Indian sample. *Forensic Sci. Med. Pathol.* **2012**, *8*, 94–100. [CrossRef]
29. Filho, I.E.M.; Lopez-Capp, T.T.; Biazevic, M.G.H.; Michel-Crosato, E. Sexual dimorphism using odontometric indexes: Analysis of three statistical techniques. *J. Forensic Leg. Med.* **2016**, *44*, 37–42. [CrossRef]
30. Filipovic, G.; Kanjevac, T.; Cetenovic, B.; Ajdukovic, Z.; Petrovic, N. Sexual dimorphism in the dimensions of teeth in serbian population. *Coll. Antropol.* **2016**, *40*, 23–28. Available online: http://www.ncbi.nlm.nih.gov/pubmed/27301233 (accessed on 7 May 2020).
31. Bolton, W.A. Disharmony in tooth size and its relation to the analysis and treatment of malocclusion. *Angle Orthod.* **1985**, *28*, 113–130.
32. Machado, V.; Botelho, J.; Amaral, A.; Proença, L.; Alves, R.; Rua, J.; Cavacas, M.A.; Delgado, A.S.; Mendes, J.J. Prevalence and extent of chronic periodontitis and its risk factors in a Portuguese subpopulation: A retrospective cross-sectional study and analysis of Clinical Attachment Loss. *PeerJ* **2018**, *6*, e5258. [CrossRef] [PubMed]
33. Botelho, J.; Machado, V.; Proença, L.; Alves, R.; Cavacas, M.A.; Amaro, L.; Mendes, J.J. Study of Periodontal Health in Almada-Seixal (SoPHiAS): A cross-sectional study in the Lisbon Metropolitan Area. *Sci. Rep.* **2019**, *9*, 1–10. [CrossRef] [PubMed]

© 2020 by the authors. Licensee MDPI, Basel, Switzerland. This article is an open access article distributed under the terms and conditions of the Creative Commons Attribution (CC BY) license (http://creativecommons.org/licenses/by/4.0/).

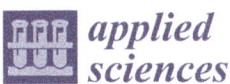

Article

Comparison of Pain Perception between Clear Aligners and Fixed Appliances: A Systematic Review and Meta-Analysis

Dinis Pereira [1,2], Vanessa Machado [1,2,*], João Botelho [2], Luís Proença [3], José João Mendes [2] and Ana Sintra Delgado [1,2]

1. Orthodontics Department, CRU, CiiEM, Egas Moniz–Cooperativa de Ensino Superior, 2829-511 Almada, Portugal; adtper@gmail.com (D.P.); anasintradelgado@gmail.com (A.S.D.)
2. Clinical Research Unit (CRU), Centro de Investigação Interdisciplinar Egas Moniz (CiiEM), Instituto Universitário Egas Moniz, 2829-511 Almada, Portugal; jbotelho@egasmoniz.edu.pt (J.B.); jmendes@egasmoniz.edu.pt (J.J.M.)
3. Quantitative Methods for Health Research Unit (MQIS), CiiEM, Egas Moniz—Cooperativa de Ensino Superior, 2829-511 Almada, Portugal; lproenca@egasmoniz.edu.pt
* Correspondence: vmachado@egasmoniz.edu.pt

Received: 23 May 2020; Accepted: 19 June 2020; Published: 22 June 2020

Featured Application: Clear aligners are associated with significantly less pain than fixed appliances during the first seven days of orthodontic treatment.

Abstract: We aimed to compare the pain discomfort levels between clear aligners and fixed appliances at multiple time points. Four electronic databases (Pubmed, Medline, CENTRAL and Scholar) were searched up to May 2020. There were no year or language restrictions. Randomized clinical trials and case–control studies comparing pain perception through pain visual analog scale (VAS) in patients treated with clear aligners and with fixed appliances were included. Risk of bias within and across studies was assessed using Cochrane tool and Newcastle–Ottawa Scale (NOS) approach. Random-effects meta-analysis were conducted. VAS score and analgesic consumption were collected. Random-effects meta-analyses were used to synthesize available data. Following the review protocol, five articles met the inclusion criteria and were included, with a total of 273 participants (177 females, 96 males). Overall, clear aligners were associated with significantly less pain than fixed appliances during the first seven days of orthodontic treatment. Patients treated with clear aligners experience less pain discomfort than those treated with fixed appliances and consume less analgesics, with SORT A recommendation.

Keywords: clear aligners; fixed appliances; pain perception; VAS (visual analog scale) scale; systematic review; meta-analysis

1. Introduction

With the increase of esthetic requirements, facial's micro and macro-esthetic and smile have become a priority for adolescents and adults [1,2]. Consequently, patients lean to more esthetic and comfortable orthodontic treatments [3].

In 1945, Kesling introduced the concept of clear aligners, that aimed to stress minor tooth movement, usually at the end of orthodontic treatment or to treat minor alignment relapse [4]. Since 1998, clear aligners have become popular and quickly the preferred orthodontic appliances for patients with high esthetic demands [5,6]. In addition, mechanical tooth movement is associated with cognitive, affective and behavioral responses [7] and periodontal mechanoreceptors and chewing muscles (as source of pain receptors) also contribute to pain experience [8,9].

Clear aligners are esthetically more appealing than fixed appliances with brackets and wires [1] and patients benefit by being able to have full access to remove clear aligners to eat and for oral hygiene. Still, patients treated with clear aligners have better periodontal health than those with fixed appliances, and they promote better compliance with oral hygiene in teenagers [10–12].

Moreover, pain experience after initial archwire placement in fixed appliances is well established, comparing multistrand stainless steel and superelastic NiTi archwires [13–20]. However, the difference in the pain perception of clear aligners compared with fixed appliances remains unclear. A recent systematic review concluded that orthodontic patients treated with Invisalign appear to feel lower levels of pain than those treated with fixed appliances during the first few days of treatment, however they were not able to synthetize the magnitude of this difference [21].

Patients choose clear aligners in hope that these appliances will have low impact on their quality of life [22]. Therefore, it becomes relevant to evaluate whether there is a difference in pain perception between fixed appliances and clear aligners. In this sense, we may contribute to a more grounded decision by the patient and the clinician.

Our main objective in this systematic review was to compare the discomfort levels between clear aligners and fixed appliances. Second, we analyzed analgesic consumption difference between the aforementioned orthodontic appliances. The review PICO research question is "Do clear aligners have less pain discomfort impact than fixed appliances treatment in orthodontic patients?", with the following statements: orthodontic patients (patients—P); clear aligners (intervention/exposure—I); fixed appliances (comparison—C); pain discomfort (outcome—O). Our null hypothesis was that clear aligners cause similar pain perception than conventional fixed appliances.

2. Materials and Methods

2.1. Subsection

The present systematic review was conducted and reported according to the preferred reporting items for systematic reviews and meta-analyses (PRISMA) guidelines for reporting studies that evaluate health care interventions [23] (in detail in Supplementary Table S1) and its extension for abstracts [24]. The protocol was previously defined and has been registered in the International Prospective Register of Systematic Reviews (PROSPERO; CRD42019124534).

2.2. Eligibility Criteria

Studies were eligible for inclusion based on the following criteria:

1. Clear aligners treatment comparing with fixed appliances and determined pain discomfort through pain visual analog scale (VAS) at multiple time points;
2. Randomized and non-randomized studies;
3. Studies in humans.

The exclusion criteria were:

1. Studies reporting results emerging from questionnaires;
2. Studies lacking control;
3. Retrospective studies;
4. In vitro and animal studies;
5. Case reports/case series;
6. Editorials, opinions, narrative reviews and technique description articles, without reported sample.

2.3. Search Strategy

A total of four electronic databases (Pubmed, Medline, CENTRAL and Google Scholar) were searched systematically until May 2020. The strategy used for the electronic search was the following:

(VAS OR visual analog scale OR VAS scale OR pain perception OR pain) AND (Invisalign OR Invisalign aligner OR clear aligner) AND (orthodontic brackets OR bracket OR fixed appliance). The reference lists of included articles and relevant reviews were manually searched. Gray literature was searched using the latter strategy in OpenGray (www.opengrey.eu).

2.4. Assessment of Validity

The eligibility of each study was assessed independently by two investigators (VM and DP), who screened the titles and/or abstracts of retrieved studies. Inclusion was dependent on the following eligibility criteria: randomized clinical trials and case–control studies who compare the discomfort level produced by fixed appliances and clear aligners at multiple time points. Final selection of studies was performed by three authors independently (VM, DP, JB) and verified by a fourth and fifth author (JJM, ASD), by reviewing the full text based on inclusion criteria above. Discussion resolved any disagreements. Non-full papers, such as conference abstracts, thesis and letters to editors, were excluded.

2.5. Data Extraction

Characteristics of the included studies and numerical data were extracted in duplicate by two authors (VM and DP) onto a predefined data extraction table: citation, publication status and year of publication, study design, setting, number of cases and characteristics of the participants (mean age, sex), VAS scores at multiple time points, type of fixed appliances and analgesic consumption. Final data were reviewed by a third author (JB).

2.6. Risk of Bias of Included Studies

Risk of bias (RoB) was performed by two independent reviewers (VM and JB). In areas of disagreements, a collective decision was obtained after a discussion between all authors to approach a consensus, with an opinion of a third reviewer (DP). RoB of RCTs was assessed with the Cochrane RoB2 tool [25]. Case–control and cohort studies were appraised with the Newcastle–Ottawa scale. "Stars" (points) were attributed for each methodologic quality criterion and each study could achieve a maximum of 8 points. Studies with 7 to 8 points (80% or more of the domains satisfactorily fulfilled) were arbitrarily considered to be of low RoB, studies with 5 to 6 stars were of medium RoB and studies with less than 5 stars were of high RoB. Disagreements between the review authors over the risk of bias in particular studies were resolved by discussion, with the involvement of a third review author (DP) where necessary.

2.7. Summary Measures & Synthesis of Results

For the conversion of median and interquartile range VAS score values to mean and standard deviations, Hozo et al. [26] procedure was used, under the assumption of normal distribution. All statistical analyses were performed in R version 3.4.1 (R Studio Team 2018, Boston, MA, USA) using a DerSimonian–Laird random-effects model [27]. All random-effects meta-analysis and forest plots were performed using 'meta' package [28].

First, pain discomfort through VAS score of clear aligners versus fixed appliances was appraised through DerSimonian–Laird (DS) random-effect analysis. Of the included studies, the percentage of analgesic consumption was also carried out, through binary random-effects analysis. Quantity I^2 was used to measure to account for homogeneity and calculated through the χ^2 test. Publication bias analysis was planned to be performed if, at least, we had 10 or more studies included [29]. All tests are two-tailed with alpha set at 0.05, except for the homogeneity test whose significance level cutoff will consider to be 0.10 due to the low power of the χ^2 test with a limited amount of studies.

2.8. Strength of Recommendation

The SORT (strength of recommendation taxonomy) was used to judge the strength and quality of the evidence [30]. We discussed the outcomes of the present systematic review, clinical recommendations and future necessary research.

3. Results

3.1. Study Selection

From the databases and other sources, the initial search resulted in a total of 98 record, resulting in 58 after duplicates removal. Following title and abstract screening, 23 studies were selected for full-text evaluation. Nevertheless, after full-text eligibility assessment, 18 studies were excluded (in detail in Supplementary Table S2). Therefore, the meta-analysis was performed on the basis of 5 articles. The flow chart of study selection together with reasons for exclusion is provided in Figure 1.

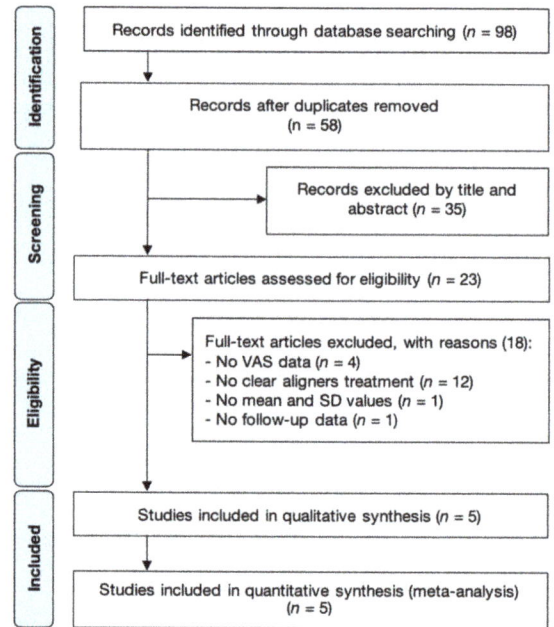

Figure 1. PRISMA (preferred reporting items for systematic reviews and meta-analyses) flowchart.

3.2. Study Characteristics

Three prospective studies evaluated the pain discomfort of clear aligners through the comparison with fixed appliances. A total of 273 participants (177 females, 96 males) were included. The characteristic of the participants is shown in Table 1.

Table 1. Included studies characteristics.

Study	Country	N (F/M)	Participants CA	Participants FA	Outcome	Funding
Miller (2007) [31]	USA	60 (43/17)	33	27	Adults treated with Invisalign aligners experienced less pain and fewer negative impacts on their lives during the first week of orthodontic treatment than did those treated with fixed appliances	NR
Shalish (2012) [32]	USA	68 (45/23)	21	47	The Invisalign patients complained of relatively high levels of pain in the first days after insertion; however this group was characterized by the lowest level of oral symptoms and by a similar level of general activity disturbances and oral dysfunction compared to the Buccal appliance.	NR
White (2017) [6]	USA	41 (24/17)	23	18	Patients treated with traditional fixed appliances reported greater discomfort and consumed more analgesics than patients treated with aligners.	Partially funded by the Robert E. Gaylord Endowed Chair in Orthodontics and by Align Technology
Almasoud (2018) [33]	Saudi Arabia	64 (42/22)	32	32	During the first week of orthodontic treatment, patients treated with Invisalign aligners reported lower pain than did those treated with passive self-ligating fixed appliances.	NR
Piergentili (2019) [34]	Italy	40 (23/17)	20	20	Therapy with traditional fixed orthodontics appliances caused more discomfort to the patients, than clear aligner therapy	NR

CA—clear aligners; FA—fixed appliances; USA—United States of America; NR—not reported.

3.3. Risk of Bias within Studies

One RCT was included and was assessed as having some concerns of risk of bias [6] (Figure 2). Table 2 (NOS scale scores) shows the risk of bias assessment for the included studies and all four studies were considered of low risk of bias [31–34].

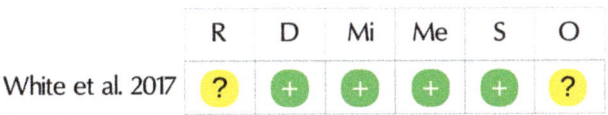

Figure 2. RoB2 assessment. R—bias arising from the randomization process; D—bias due to deviations from intended interventions; Mi—bias due to missing outcome data; Me—bias in measurement of the outcome; S—bias in selection of the reported result; O—overall risk of bias.

Table 2. NOS (Newcastle–Ottawa Scale) score for case–control studies.

	Selection				Comparability	Outcome			TOTAL	
	1	2	3	4	5	6	7	8		Score
Miller (2007) [31]	a	a	a	a	a	a	a	a	8	Low
Shalish (2012) [32]	a	a	a	a	a	a	a	a	8	Low
Almasoud (2018) [33]	c	a	a	a	a	a	a	a	7	Low
Piergentili (2019) [34]	a	a	a	a	a	a	a	a	8	Low

1-case definition adequacy; 2-representativeness of the cases; 3-selection of controls; 4-definition of controls; 5-comparability of cohorts on the basis of the design or analysis; 6-ascertainment of outcome; 7-save method of ascertainment for cases and controls; 8-nonresponse rate.

3.4. Synthesis of Results

Data from three studies including 273 patients reported pain discomfort through VAS score of clear aligners versus fixed appliances [6,31–34]. Four studies provided data on a daily basis [6,31,32,34], while one had data for pain discomfort at day 1, 3 and 7 after [33].

Clear aligners promote lower pain experience than patients using fixed appliances, and the difference is statistically significant for 1, 3, 6 and 7 days of follow-up (Table 3). The overall pain experience also favored clear aligners. Funnel plot analysis revealed no publication bias (Figure 3).

Table 3. Subgroup meta-analysis of VAS score from 1 to 7 days of follow-up.

Subgroup Meta-Analysis	n	MD	95% CI	p-Value	I² (%)	Tau	p-Value
Day 1	6	1.07	(0.00; 2.13)	<0.001	84.9	1.16	<0.001
Day 2	5	0.60	(−0.20; 1.41)	>0.05	80.7	0.77	<0.001
Day 3	6	1.25	(0.32; 2.17)	<0.001	83.0	0.99	<0.001
Day 4	5	0.79	(−0.07; 1.65)	>0.05	83.8	0.84	<0.001
Day 5	5	0.62	(−0.13; 1.37)	>0.05	83.7	0.71	<0.001
Day 6	5	0.76	(0.31; 1.21)	<0.001	67.6	0.38	<0.001
Day 7	6	0.79	(0.37; 1.22)	<0.001	64.2	0.36	<0.001
Overall	6	0.33	(0.45; 1.57)	<0.001	80.5	0.58	<0.001

Test for subgroup differences (random effects model): Q = 1.62, p = 0.9514. MD–Mean Difference.

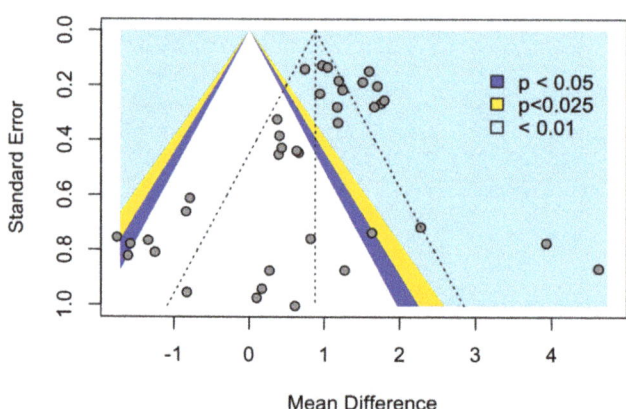

Figure 3. Funnel plot. The outer dashed lines indicate the triangular region within which 95% of studies are expected to lie in the absence of both biases and heterogeneity (fixed effect summary log odds ratio ± 1.96 × standard error of summary log odds ratio). The dashed vertical line corresponds to no intervention effect. The distribution gives a clear visual impression of symmetry, which is confirmed by a $p > 0.05$.

A detailed number of analgesic consumption at day 1, 3 and 7 after, were reported in three studies [6,31,33]. Overall, patients treated with clear aligners have significantly less analgesic consumption compared with fixed appliances group control, one day and seven days after treatment beginning (Table 4). Overall, patients with fixed appliances consume more analgesics at the beginning of treatment.

Table 4. Subgroup meta-analysis of Analgesic consumption at 1, 3 and 7 days of follow-up.

Subgroup Meta-Analysis	n	OR	95% CI	p-Value	I² (%)	Tau	p-Value
Day 1	3	0.15	(0.04; 0.50)	<0.001	84.9	49.3	0.14
Day 3	3	0.75	(0.11; 5.10)	<0.001	83.0	81.0	<0.001
Day 7	3	0.23	(0.52; 0.99)	<0.001	64.2	0.0	0.79
Overall	3	0.30	(0.12; 0.72)	<0.001	80.5	58.8	0.01

Test for subgroup differences (random effects model): Q = 1.97, p = 0.3734. OR–Odds Ratio.

3.5. Synthesis of Results

According to the SORT recommendation, the evidence revealed that clear aligners produce less pain experience than fixed appliances, based on consistent findings of at least two good-quality meta-analyses that obtained significant results (SORT A) [30].

4. Discussion

4.1. Summary of Main Findings

This systematic review demonstrate that clear aligners are significantly associated with less pain rather than fixed appliances during the first week of orthodontic treatment, with an overall SORT A recommendation. Clear aligners patients present less risk of analgesics consumption compared to patients with fixed appliances and present significant differences.

4.2. Quality of the Evidence, Limitations and Potential Biases in the Review Process

The strengths of this systematic review include the extensive unrestrictive literature search, with a rigorous and predetermined protocol implemented in each phase. However, there are limitations worth to mention among the included studies.

The included investigations were of small samples, and one of them lack sample size calculation [31]. As well, there are a diversity of fixed appliances description since one did not refer the type of buccal fixed appliances [31], one used self-ligated fixed appliance [33], three used a twin-bracket fixed appliance [6], and one also had lingual brackets [32,34]. Though passive self-ligating systems result in minor periodontal ligament ischemia and therefore less discomfort [35], literature evidences that pain experience in the beginning of treatment is independent of bracket type [36–38]. The type and size of archwires were described in four studies [6], though they differed in type and size among them, which is also a limitation worth mentioning. Nevertheless, previous studies have found no significant differences in the pain perception using different archwires types [36,39,40]. Furthermore, Piergentilli et al. [33] have placed the fixed appliance exclusively in the maxillary arch during the first week of treatment, and this may explain also the observed heterogeneity.

Moreover, only one study [6] performed random selection, while the remaining four [31–34] did not randomly assigned the treatment modalities due to their cohort design nature. However, randomizing adult patients is not simple, since some of whom are unwilling or unable to comply with the random assignment due to esthetic reasons [32]. This difficulty limits the ability to completely randomize the study. The fact that the patient has a choice demonstrates personality traits, which can impair the perception of pain. Notwithstanding, the RCT included in this review [33] lacked allocation concealment contributing to the overall concern on the risk of bias [33]. Allocation concealment is predictably difficult to achieve in this type of studies in which the intervention is a removable appliance and its control a fixed appliance.

Additionally, pain experience is a notoriously subjective response and there is a nonlinear relationship upon multiple factors such as age, gender, individual pain threshold, the magnitude of the force applied, present emotional state and stress, cultural differences and previous pain experiences [14,17,19,41–44]. A hypothetical limitation would be the fact that there is an unbalanced gender ratio. However, gender has no significant effect on orthodontic pain perception [14,17,19,45], except in adolescents, where females have less pain tolerance than males [46,47].

Finally, placing attachments at the beginning of the clear aligner treatment is relevant for pain perception because they cause more pressure during the insertion of the aligner. Among the included studies, Miller et al. [31] did not place attachments, two studies used attachments since they placed the first aligners [6] and Almasoud [33] delayed the attachments placement until the third set of aligners. Despite Shalish et al. [33] did not refer the placement of attachments, patients with clear aligners reported more pain than those using buccal fixed appliances, and alike those using lingual fixed appliances patients. The reason to this pain experience difference could be a greater mechanical force caused by the attachment placement, though they should be investigated deeply in the future. In addition, the importance of the periodontal mechanoreceptors and chewing muscles during clear aligners tooth movement is a matter to be further investigated.

5. Conclusions

Within the limitations of this systematic review, the results show that patients treated with clear aligners experience less pain and discomfort than patients treated with fixed appliances. This information may clarify patients about what to expect during the beginning of orthodontic treatment. In the future, larger randomized clinical trials are needed to demonstrate unequivocally that clear aligners are more comfortable than fixed appliances throughout orthodontics treatment.

Implications for Clinical Practice and Research

These findings may help both patients and clinicians in the treatment modality decision, concerning pain parameters and analgesic consultation, in the first phase of orthodontic treatment.

In the main, randomized clinical trials are needed to perform a robust comparison of clear aligners and buccal fixed appliances. Aspects concerning long-term outcomes appraisal, objective measurements of patient-centered reported outcomes (such as quality of life) and adverse effects (including allergies, periodontal damages and functional impairment) are important factors to consider.

Additionally, the present review encompassed mainly Invisalign® aligners. Future research should be conducted in different clear aligners systems, to find out if exists significant differences between different types of clear aligners systems in pain perception and analgesic drugs intake.

Supplementary Materials: The following are available online at http://www.mdpi.com/2076-3417/10/12/4276/s1, Table S1: PRISMA Checklist, Table S2: List of potentially relevant studies not included in the systematic review, along with the reasons for exclusion.

Author Contributions: Conceptualization, D.P., V.M., J.B., L.P., J.J.M., A.S.D.; methodology, V.M. and J.B.; software, V.M. and J.B.; validation D.P., V.M. and J.B.; formal analysis, J.B.; data curation, D.P., V.M. and J.B. All authors have read and agreed to the published version of the manuscript.

Funding: This research received no external funding.

Conflicts of Interest: The authors declare no conflict of interest.

References

1. Ziuchkovski, J.P.; Fields, H.W.; Johnston, W.M.; Lindsey, D.T. Assessment of perceived orthodontic appliance attractiveness. *Am. J. Orthod. Dentofac. Orthop.* **2008**, *133*, 68–78. [CrossRef] [PubMed]
2. Sarver, D.M. Interactions of hard tissues, soft tissues, and growth over time, and their impact on orthodontic diagnosis and treatment planning. *Am. J. Orthod. Dentofac. Orthop.* **2015**, *148*, 380–386. [CrossRef]
3. Rosvall, M.D.; Fields, H.W.; Ziuchkovski, J.; Rosenstiel, S.F.; Johnston, W.M. Attractiveness, acceptability, and value of orthodontic appliances. *Am. J. Orthod. Dentofac. Orthop.* **2009**, *135*, e1–e276. [CrossRef]
4. Kesling, H.D. The philosophy of the tooth positioning appliance. *Am. J. Orthod. Oral Surg.* **1945**, *31*, 297–304. [CrossRef]
5. Wong, B.H.; Scholz, R.P.; Turpin, D.L. Invisalign A to Z. *Am. J. Orthod. Dentofac. Orthop.* **2002**, *121*, 540–541. [CrossRef]

6. White, D.W.; Julien, K.C.; Jacob, H.; Campbell, P.M.; Buschang, P.H. Discomfort associated with Invisalign and traditional brackets: A randomized, prospective trial. *Angle Orthod.* **2017**, *87*, 801–808. [CrossRef]
7. Giddon, D.B.; Anderson, N.K.; Will, L.A. Cognitive, Affective, and Behavioral Responses Associated with Mechanical Tooth Movement. *Semin. Orthod.* **2007**, *13*, 212–219. [CrossRef]
8. Piancino, M.G.; Isola, G.; Cannavale, R.; Cutroneo, G.; Vermiglio, G.; Bracco, P.; Anastasi, G.P. From periodontal mechanoreceptors to chewing motor control: A systematic review. *Arch. Oral Biol.* **2017**, *78*, 109–121. [CrossRef]
9. Isola, G.; Anastasi, G.P.; Matarese, G.; Williams, R.C.; Cutroneo, G.; Bracco, P.; Piancino, M.G. Functional and molecular outcomes of the human masticatory muscles. *Oral Dis.* **2018**, *24*, 1428–1441. [CrossRef]
10. Abbate, G.M.; Caria, M.P.; Montanari, P.; Mannu, C.; Orrù, G.; Caprioglio, A.; Levrini, L. Parodontale Gesundheit von Teenagern mit herausnehmbaren Alignern und festsitzenden kieferorthopädischen Apparaturen. *J. Orofac. Orthop.* **2015**, *76*, 240–250. [CrossRef]
11. Azaripour, A.; Weusmann, J.; Mahmoodi, B.; Peppas, D.; Gerhold-Ay, A.; Van Noorden, C.J.F.; Willershausen, B. Braces versus Invisalign®: Gingival parameters and patients' satisfaction during treatment: A cross-sectional study. *BMC Oral Health* **2015**, *15*, 1–5. [CrossRef] [PubMed]
12. Lu, H.; Tang, H.; Zhou, T.; Kang, N. Assessment of the periodontal health status in patients undergoing orthodontic treatment with fixed appliances and Invisalign system. *Medicine* **2018**, *97*, e0248. [CrossRef] [PubMed]
13. Wang, Y.; Liu, C.; Jian, F.; Mcintyre, G.T.; Millett, D.T.; Hickman, J.; Lai, W. Initial arch wires used in orthodontic treatment with fixed appliances. *Cochrane Database Syst. Rev.* **2018**, *7*. [CrossRef] [PubMed]
14. Wilson, S.; Ngan, P.; Kess, B. Time course of the discomfort in young patients undergoing orthodontic treatment. *Pediatr. Dent.* **1989**, *11*, 107–110. [PubMed]
15. Jones, M.; Chan, C. The pain and discomfort experienced during orthodntic treatment: A randomized controlled clinical trial of two intial aligning arch wires. *Am. J. Orthod. Dentofac. Orthop.* **1992**, *102*, 373–381. [CrossRef]
16. Ngan, P.; Kess, B.; Wilson, S. Perception of discomfort by patients undergoing orthodontic treatment. *Am. J. Orthod. Dentofac. Orthop.* **1989**, *96*, 47–53. [CrossRef]
17. Scheurer, P.A.; Firestone, A.R.; Bürgin, W.B. Perception of pain as a result of orthodontic treatment with fixed appliances. *Eur. J. Orthod.* **1996**, *18*, 349–357. [CrossRef]
18. Stewart, F.N.; Kerr, W.J.S.; Taylor, P.J.S. Appliance wear: The patient's point of view. *Eur. J. Orthod.* **1997**, *19*, 377–382. [CrossRef]
19. Krishnan, V.; Davidovitch, Z. Cellular, molecular, and tissue-level reactions to orthodontic force. *Am. J. Orthod. Dentofac. Orthop.* **2006**, *129*, e1–e469. [CrossRef]
20. Grieve, W.G.; Johnson, G.K.; Moore, R.N.; Reinhardt, R.A.; DuBois, L.M. Prostaglandin E (PGE) and interleukin-1β (IL-1β) levels in gingival crevicular fluid during human orthodontic tooth movement. *Am. J. Orthod. Dentofac. Orthop.* **1994**, *105*, 369–374. [CrossRef]
21. Cardoso, P.C.; Espinosa, D.G.; Mecenas, P.; Flores-Mir, C.; Normando, D. Pain level between clear aligners and fixed appliances: A systematic review. *Prog. Orthod.* **2020**, *21*, 3. [CrossRef]
22. Flores-Mir, C.; Brandelli, J.; Pacheco-Pereira, C. Patient satisfaction and quality of life status after 2 treatment modalities: Invisalign and conventional fixed appliances. *Am. J. Orthod. Dentofac. Orthop.* **2018**, *154*, 639–644. [CrossRef] [PubMed]
23. Liberati, A.; Altman, D.G.; Tetzlaff, J.; Mulrow, C.; Gøtzsche, P.C.; Ioannidis, J.P.A.; Clarke, M.; Devereaux, P.J.; Kleijnen, J.; Moher, D. The PRISMA statement for reporting systematic reviews and meta-analyses of studies that evaluate health care interventions: Explanation and elaboration. *PLoS Med.* **2009**, *6*, e1000100. [CrossRef] [PubMed]
24. Beller, E.M.; Glasziou, P.P.; Altman, D.G.; Hopewell, S.; Bastian, H.; Chalmers, I.; Gøtzsche, P.C.; Lasserson, T.; Tovey, D. PRISMA for Abstracts: Reporting Systematic Reviews in Journal and Conference Abstracts. *PLoS Med.* **2013**, *10*, e1001419. [CrossRef]
25. Sterne, J.A.C.; Savović, J.; Page, M.J.; Elbers, R.G.; Blencowe, N.S.; Boutron, I.; Cates, C.J.; Cheng, H.Y.; Corbett, M.S.; Eldridge, S.M.; et al. RoB 2: A revised tool for assessing risk of bias in randomised trials. *BMJ* **2019**, *366*, 1–8. [CrossRef] [PubMed]
26. Hozo, S.P.; Djulbegovic, B.; Hozo, I. Estimating the mean and variance from the median, range, and the size of a sample. *BMC Med. Res. Methodol.* **2005**, *5*, 1–10. [CrossRef]

27. Schwarzer, G.; Carpenter, J.R.; Rücker, G. *Meta-Analysis with R*; Springer: Berlin/Heidelberg, Germany, 2015; ISBN 9783319214153.
28. Schwarzer, G. Meta: An R Package for Meta-Analysis. *R News* **2007**, *7*, 40–45.
29. Higgins, J.; Green, S. Cochrane Handbook for Systematic Reviews of Interventions; 5.1.0 (updated March 2011); The Cochrane Collaboration: 2011. Available online: https://www.cochrane-handbook.org (accessed on 15 April 2020).
30. Newman, M.G.; Weyant, R.; Hujoel, P. JEBDP Improves Grading System and Adopts Strength of Recommendation Taxonomy Grading (SORT) for Guidelines and Systematic Reviews. *J. Evid. Based. Dent. Pract.* **2007**, *7*, 147–150. [CrossRef]
31. Miller, K.B.; McGorray, S.P.; Womack, R.; Quintero, J.C.; Perelmuter, M.; Gibson, J.; Dolan, T.A.; Wheeler, T.T. A comparison of treatment impacts between Invisalign aligner and fixed appliance therapy during the first week of treatment. *Am. J. Orthod. Dentofac. Orthop.* **2007**, *131*, e1–e302. [CrossRef]
32. Shalish, M.; Cooper-Kazaz, R.; Ivgi, I.; Canetti, L.; Tsur, B.; Bachar, E.; Chaushu, S. Adult patients' adjustability to orthodontic appliances. Part I: A comparison between Labial, Lingual, and Invisalign^{TM}. *Eur. J. Orthod.* **2012**, *34*, 724–730. [CrossRef]
33. Almasoud, N.N. Pain perception among patients treated with passive self-ligating fixed appliances and invisalign®aligners during the first week of orthodontic treatment. *Korean J. Orthod.* **2018**, *48*, 326–332. [CrossRef] [PubMed]
34. Piergentili, M.; Bucci, R.; Madariaga, A.C.P.; Martina, S.; Rongo, R.; D'Antò, V. Pain and discomfort associated with labial multibracket appliances vs clear aligners. *J. Aligner Orthod.* **2019**, *3*, 205–212.
35. Wright, N.; Modarai, F.; Cobourne, M.T.; DiBiase, A.T. Do you do Damon ®? What is the current evidence base underlying the philosophy of this appliance system? *J. Orthod.* **2011**, *38*, 222–230. [CrossRef] [PubMed]
36. Fleming, P.S.; DiBiase, A.T.; Sarri, G.; Lee, R.T. Pain experience during initial alignment with a self-ligating and a conventional fixed orthodontic appliance system. *Angle Orthod.* **2009**, *79*, 46–50. [CrossRef]
37. Fleming, P.S.; Johal, A. Self-ligating brackets in orthodontics a systematic review. *Angle Orthod.* **2010**, *80*, 575–584. [CrossRef] [PubMed]
38. Miles, P.G.; Weyant, R.J.; Rustveld, L. A clinical trial of damon 2^{TM} Vs conventional twin brackets during initial alignment. *Angle Orthod.* **2006**, *76*, 480–485.
39. Rahman, S.; Spencer, R.J.; Littlewood, S.J.; O'Dywer, L.; Barber, S.K.; Russell, J.S. A multicenter randomized controlled trial to compare a self-ligating bracket with a conventional bracket in a UK population: Part 2: Pain perception. *Angle Orthod.* **2016**, *86*, 149–156. [CrossRef]
40. Scott, P.; Sherriff, M.; DiBiase, A.T.; Cobourne, M.T. Perception of discomfort during initial orthodontic tooth alignment using a self-ligating or conventional bracket system: A randomized clinical trial. *Eur. J. Orthod.* **2008**, *30*, 227–232. [CrossRef]
41. Bergius, M.; Kiliaridis, S.; Berggren, U. Pain in orthodontics. A review and discussion of the literature. *J. Orofac. Orthop.* **2000**, *61*, 125–137. [CrossRef]
42. Firestone, A.R.; Scheurer, P.A.; Bürgin, W.B. Patients' anticipation of pain and pain-related side effects, and their perception of pain as a result of orthodontic treatment with fixed appliances. *Eur. J. Orthod.* **1999**, *21*, 387–396. [CrossRef]
43. Brown, D.F.; Moerenhout, R.G. The pain experience and psychological adjustment to orthodontic treatment of preadolescents, adolescents, and adults. *Am. J. Orthod. Dentofac. Orthop.* **1991**, *100*, 349–356. [CrossRef]
44. Chow, J.; Cioffi, I. Pain and orthodontic patient compliance: A clinical perspective. *Semin. Orthod.* **2018**, *24*, 242–247. [CrossRef]
45. Erdinç, A.; Dinçer, B. Perception of pain during orthodontic treatment with fixed appliances. *Eur. J. Orthod.* **2004**, *26*, 79–85. [CrossRef] [PubMed]
46. Sandhu, S.S.; Sandhu, J. Orthodontic pain: An interaction between age and sex in early and middle adolescence. *Angle Orthod.* **2013**, *83*, 966–972. [CrossRef] [PubMed]
47. Alhaija, E.S.A.; AlDaikki, A.; Al-Omairi, M.K.; Al-Khateeb, S.N. The relationship between personality traits, pain perception and attitude toward orthodontic treatment. *Angle Orthod.* **2010**, *80*, 1141–1149. [CrossRef]

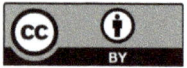

© 2020 by the authors. Licensee MDPI, Basel, Switzerland. This article is an open access article distributed under the terms and conditions of the Creative Commons Attribution (CC BY) license (http://creativecommons.org/licenses/by/4.0/).

MDPI
St. Alban-Anlage 66
4052 Basel
Switzerland
Tel. +41 61 683 77 34
Fax +41 61 302 89 18
www.mdpi.com

Applied Sciences Editorial Office
E-mail: applsci@mdpi.com
www.mdpi.com/journal/applsci

www.ingramcontent.com/pod-product-compliance
Lightning Source LLC
LaVergne TN
LVHW070544100526
838202LV00012B/375